D1496791

ERRATA

Following publication of "A DIABETIC PARTY COOKBOOK by the 3 Aunts" the authors learned that the artificial sweetener "Sucaryl" is no longer manufactured in the granulated or powdered form. Liquid Sucaryl, however, is still available. For the granulated Sucaryl called for in a number of recipes, any one of several granulated artificial sweeteners may be substituted on an equal-measure basis (cup-for-cup, tablespoon-for-tablespoon). Included in these are the granulated forms of Sug'r Like, Sprinkle Sweet, Sugar Twin, and Sweetness and Light. Also, granulated or powdered Sweet'n Low and liquid Sucaryl may be substituted but in reduced measure, namely, 1/8 teaspoon of either preparation in place of 1 teaspoon of granulated or powdered Sucaryl.

A DIABETIC
Party
COOKBOOK

A DIABETIC

Party

COOKBOOK

by the

3 Aunts

Betty Lou Nelson
Margaret Hippen, M.S., R.D.
Jane Ewan

Booklore Publishers, Inc.
P.O. Drawer 3679, Sarasota, FL 33578

IV

ISBN 0-931110-01-7

Library of Congress Catalog Card Number: 79-53199
Printed in the United States of America

PREFACE

It's time for a party! This means having your favorite people in for fun and food so interesting that you won't think about diets. Remember, a successful party does not just happen. You have to plan it, and we will show you how.

This Diabetic Party Cookbook offers a challenge to those of you who entertain in households where diabetes must be considered. It has been written in answer to complaints that there is no party cookbook for diabetics, that cooking for these people is dull and uninspired. But there is no reason why the diabetic child, teenager, or adult cannot enjoy a variety of fun, food, and parties—so take a positive approach and start planning.

Within this book we have presented a choice of interesting menus and party ideas for all age groups. You will find them excellent guidelines in helping to make diabetic cooking creative.

The book is not designed to give medical advice, but the party programs and recipes have been developed through cooperation with and with the approval of registered dietitians.

Special thanks for encouragement and support are extended to two associates: Macarita Young, M.S., R.D., who is a research nutritionist, a special therapeutic consultant, and a professor of nutrition; and Phyllis Heald, well-known writer, who sparked the idea for the book and made valuable suggestions.

The Three Aunts—
Betty Lou Nelson
Margaret Hippen, M.S., R.D.
Jane Ewan

CONTENTS

INTRODUCTION

The Diabetic Exchange System, briefly outlined on the following pages, has been used throughout this book. The food exchange per serving for each recipe as well as for each menu is given. Thus the party fare can be easily fitted into the diabetic's diet plan for the day. With knowledge of the exchange system, the "Mix and Match" section (Part IV) can be used to provide additions or substitutions in a chosen menu.

The small amounts of hidden calories in these recipes are negligible and need cause no worry.

A few of the *special occasion* recipes include a very small amount of sugar. Footnotes to these recipes have been employed so that they may be easily recognized.

As an artificial sweetener, Sucaryl is designated because its sweetness has been found by the authors to be retained better during cooking than that of other similar preparations.

Sizes of meat servings refer to cooked portions and allow for weight loss in cooking processes.

DIABETIC EXCHANGE SYSTEM

The American Diabetes Association and the American Dietetic Association, in cooperation with the United States Public Health Service, have developed six "exchange lists" for the purpose of establishing uniform food values. These standard groupings of foods greatly simplify meal planning, diet prescription, and use of exchanges. They are briefly described as follows:

Milk Exchange— List 1. One exchange of milk contains 12 grams of carbohydrate, 8 grams of protein, and 10 grams of fat, and provides 170 calories. (In this book the term "Skim Milk Exchange" means a Milk Exchange *without* any Fat.)

Vegetable Exchanges— List 2A. These contain little carbohydrate or protein, and provide few calories.

Vegetable Exchanges— List 2B. One exchange contains 7 grams of carbohydrate and 2 grams of protein, and provides 36 calories.

Fruit Exchanges— List 3. One exchange of fruit (unsweetened) contains 10 grams of carbohydrate, and provides 40 calories.

Bread Exchanges— List 4. One bread exchange contains 15 grams of carbohydrate and 2 grams of protein, and provides 68 calories.

Meat Exchanges— List 5. One meat exchange contains 7 grams of protein and 5 grams of fat, and provides 73 calories.

Fat Exchanges— List 6. One fat exchange contains 5 grams of fat, and provides 45 calories.

To determine the calories contained in a specified amount of food, multiply the grams of carbohydrate by 4, the grams of protein by 4, the grams of fat by 9, and add the three products. For example: One Milk Exchange contains 12 grams of carbohydrate, 8 grams of protein, and 10 grams of fat. The calorie content is:

$$(12 \times 4) + (8 \times 4) + (10 \times 9) = 170.$$

PART I

Parties for the Diabetic

Child

Do you worry because your child goes on eating jags of hot dogs, bologna, fried chicken, hamburgers, or peanut butter? Don't let this disturb you. Such cravings are perfectly normal and in time will subside. These foods are nutritious and healthful. All you need do is accept them and work around them.

In this book we are realistic about children's eating habits and have planned menus that should be popular. All food is prepared to be served in small pieces and can be handled easily with fingers or forks.

Since it is important for diabetic children to eat regularly and not snack, well-planned menus are the answer. However, you will want to inform the mothers of your guests as to the Food Exchanges that will be served at any party.

COOKOUTS

Five menus are included for cookouts, as both boys and girls love this type of party. For a cowboy (and cowgirl) roundup the invitations can read:

> Roy Rogers (or your favorite cowboy) invites you to a real western roundup. All cowboys, cowgirls, or Indians please dress for the occasion. Check your guns with the Wagon Master or the Trail Boss. Indians please come without war paint! There will be food, fun, and lots of games.

_____(signature)
Phone number: _____
Date:_____Time: _____

With an invitation like this the children will know that they are going to have a good time. It's impossible to "brand" hamburgers or hot dogs, but an effect can be created by placing each guest's food in a grub box or chuck box made from a paper sack and labeled in crayon with his or her name.

Menus and Recipes for Four

Barbecued Little Sizzlers

> **Milk**
>
> **Barbecued Little Sizzlers**
>
> **Baked Sweet Potato**
>
> **Dill Pickle**
>
> **Tangerines**

Milk

Serve each child one 8-ounce cup of milk.
One cup equals 1 Milk Exchange.

Barbecued Little Sizzlers (4 servings—4 Sizzlers each)

16   *Little Sizzlers (small sausage links)*
12   *tablespoons Barbecue Sauce (recipe follows)*

Place sausage links on grill when charcoal is ready. Turn frequently, as they are small and will burn readily. Swab with barbecue sauce just before serving.

Barbecue Sauce (4 servings — 3 tablespoons each)

3	ounces Tomato Paste
3/4	cup hot Water
1½	tablespoons Vinegar
¼	teaspoon liquid Sucaryl
½	teaspoon Salt
1	tablespoon Worcestershire Sauce
¼	teaspoon Liquid Smoke
⅛	teaspoon Chili Powder

Mix water and tomato paste in saucepan. Add remaining ingredients. Simmer for about 1 hour.
One serving (sizzlers and sauce) equals 2 Meat Exchanges.

Baked Sweet Potatoes (4 servings — ½ cup each)

2	small Sweet Potatoes

Scrub and bake potatoes in their skins for 1 hour, at 400 degrees, in indoor oven. When done, cut each in half crosswise. Show children how to pull skins down as they eat the potato; the shell (skin) is the holder.
One serving equals 2 Bread Exchanges.

Dill Pickles (4 servings — ½ pickle each)

2	large Dill Pickles

Cut each pickle in half lengthwise.
One serving equals Zero Exchange.

Tangerines (4 servings—1 tangerine each)

    4   *large Tangerines*

Serve whole, allowing each child to peel his own fruit. One serving equals 1 Fruit Exchange.

- - - - - - - - - -

Exchanges for one serving of the entire menu equal 1 Milk, 1 Fruit, 2 Bread, 2 Meat.

* * * * *

Barbecued Shrimp

Milk

Barbecued Shrimp

Whole Green Beans   **Carrot Sticks**

French Bread

Strawberry Shortcake

Milk

Serve each child one 8-ounce cup of milk.
One cup equals 1 Milk Exchange.

Barbecued Shrimp (4 servings—5 shrimp each)

20   *medium-sized Shrimp, uncooked*

Peel and devein shrimp. Place five shrimp on each of four long skewers. Brush each side of shrimp with barbecue sauce (recipe follows). Cook over coals in grill for 3 to 4 minutes on each side.

Barbecue Sauce (4 servings—3 tablespoons each)

> 3   *ounces Tomato Paste*
> ³/₄   *cup hot Water*
> 1¹/₂ *tablespoons Vinegar*
> ¹/₄   *teaspoon liquid Sucaryl*
> ¹/₂   *teaspoon Salt*
> 1   *tablespoon Worcestershire Sauce*
> ¹/₄   *teaspoon Liquid Smoke*
> ¹/₈   *teaspoon Chili Powder*

Mix water and tomato paste in saucepan. Add remaining ingredients and simmer for about 1 hour.
One serving (shrimp and sauce) equals 1 Meat Exchange.

Whole Green Beans (4 servings—¹/₄ can each)

> 1   *can (16-ounce) Whole Green Beans*
> ¹/₄   *teaspoon Butter Flavoring*
> ¹/₄   *teaspoon Salt*

Drain beans and sprinkle with butter flavoring and salt. Serve cold.
One serving equals ¹/₂ A Vegetable Exchange.

Carrot Sticks (4 servings—3 sticks each)

> 3   *Carrots*

Scrape carrots and cut in quarters lengthwise.
One serving equals ¹/₂ B Vegetable Exchange.

French Bread (4 servings—¹/₂ slice each)

> 2   *medium-sized slices French Bread*
> 2   *teaspoons Margarine*

Cut each slice of bread in half; spread with margarine. Wrap each piece of bread in heavy foil and place on back of grill to warm while shrimp are being cooked.

One serving equals ¹/₂ Bread Exchange, ¹/₂ Fat Exchange.

Strawberry Shortcake
(4 servings — 1 biscuit plus ¹/₂ cup strawberries for each)

¹/₂   cup Biscuit Mix
¹/₈   cup Water
2   cups mashed fresh Strawberries
Granulated Sucaryl to taste

Combine biscuit mix and water; stir with fork. Divide into four equal portions and flatten into shape of biscuits. Place on cookie sheet that has been sprayed lightly with PAM. Bake in 400-degree oven for about 8 minutes.

Add granulated Sucaryl to mashed strawberries (frozen unsweetened berries may be used). Split the biscuits; cover each half biscuit with ¹/₄ cup of berries; add the other half biscuit and cover with another ¹/₄ cup of berries.

One serving equals ¹/₂ Fruit Exchange, ¹/₂ Bread Exchange.

- - - - - - - - - -

Exchanges for one serving of the entire menu equal 1 Milk, ¹/₂ A Vegetable, ¹/₂ B Vegetable, ¹/₂ Fruit, 1 Bread, 1 Meat, ¹/₂ Fat.

* * * * *

Broiled Steak

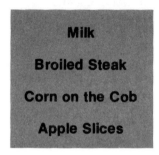

Milk

Broiled Steak

Corn on the Cob

Apple Slices

Milk

Serve each child one 8-ounce cup of milk.
One cup equals 1 Milk Exchange.

Broiled Steak (4 servings—2 ounces each)

   12   *ounces thinly sliced Fillet of Beef*

Broil beef over hot bed of coals; divide into four equal portions.
One serving equals 2 Meat Exchanges.

Corn on the Cob (4 servings—¹/₂ ear each)

   2   *medium-sized ears Corn, cut in half*
   4   *teaspoons Margarine*

Before broiling steaks, steam corn in small amount of boiling water for about 9 minutes. When corn is done, remove it from water and wrap it in foil. Place corn on back of grill to keep warm.

Melt margarine in small skillet and place on back of grill to keep it warm. Pour 1 teaspoon over each serving of corn.
One serving equals 1 Bread Exchange, 1 Fat Exchange.

Apple Slices (4 servings — ¹/₄ apple each)

Cut a large apple in quarters; remove core.
One serving equals ¹/₂ Fruit Exchange.

- - - - - - - - - -

*Exchanges for one serving of the entire menu equals 1 Milk,
¹/₂ Fruit, 1 Bread, 2 Meat, 1 Fat.*

* * * * *

Hot Dogs in Doggy Blankets

Milk

Hot Dogs in Doggy Blankets

Celery Sticks   **Tomato Wedges**

Peachy Cones

Milk

Serve each child one 8-ounce cup of milk.
One cup equals 1 Milk Exchange.

Hot Dogs in Doggy Blankets
(4 servings—2 wieners and 2 blankets each)

8   *Wieners (1 pound)*
8   *canned Biscuits*
Mustard

Roll each biscuit into an elongated shape the size of a wiener. Bake as directed for biscuits. Cool, split, and place on foil or pie tin on back of grill.

Put two wieners on each of four long skewers or roasting sticks; roast over bed of coals, turning wieners frequently. When wieners are done, make sandwiches with doggy blankets, adding mustard if desired.

One serving equals 2 Bread Exchanges, 2 Meat Exchanges.

Celery Sticks and Tomato Wedges
(4 servings—3 sticks celery and ¼ tomato for each)

3   *ribs Celery*
1   *medium-sized Tomato*

Cut each rib of celery into four sticks; divide tomato into quarters.

One serving equals 1 A Vegetable Exchange.

Peachy Cones (4 servings—1 cone each)

    4   *Ice Cream Cones*
    1   *cup Peach Jam (recipe follows)*
    1   *cup Jane's Topping**

Mix topping and jam together; divide equally among the four cones. Freeze until ready to serve.

Peach Jam (4 servings—¹/₄ cup each)

    1¹/₂   *cups water-packed Peaches*
    1¹/₂   *tablespoons granulated Sucaryl*
    1   *teaspoon Lemon Juice*
    Dash of Salt

Drain peaches well and mash. Add other ingredients. Cook slowly for about 15 minutes or until thickened. Cool thoroughly before using.

One serving (cone, jam, and topping) equals ³/₄ Fruit Exchange, ¹/₂ Bread Exchange.

- - - - - - - - - -

Exchanges for one serving of the entire menu equal 1 Milk, 1 A Vegetable, ³/₄ Fruit, 2¹/₂ Bread, 2 Meat.

* * * * *

*Use the recipe for Jane's Topping given in Part IV (see Index), but cut the amounts in half.

Hamburgers on Buns

Milk

Hamburgers on Buns

Lettuce　　　　　　　　　　　　　　　　**Onion**

Dill Pickle　　　　　　　　　　　　　　**Mustard**

Watermelon or Cantaloupe

Milk

Serve each child one 8-ounce cup of milk.
One cup equals 1 Milk Exchange.

Hamburger on Bun (4 servings — 1 hamburger each)

> ³/₄　*pound lean ground Beef*
> 4　*small Hamburger Buns*
> *Prepared Mustard*
> *Salt and Pepper*

Mix seasoning with meat, then form mixture into four patties. Flatten patties until each is a little larger than the bun. Grill hamburger meat over bed of coals. Put meat patties on buns and add mustard if desired.
One serving equals 1 Bread Exchange, 2 Meat Exchanges.

Lettuce—Dill Pickle—Sliced Onion

2   *leaves of Lettuce*
1   *Dill Pickle, sliced thin*
1/2   *medium Onion, sliced thin*

Split lettuce leaves into halves. On each half leaf put two or three slices of pickle and two or three shreds of onion. Serve with hamburgers.
One serving equals 1 A Vegetable Exchange.

Watermelon or Cantaloupe (4 servings—about 1 cup each)

4   *cups Watermelon or Cantaloupe*

Cut melons into 1/2-inch cubes. Serve in paper cups.
One serving equals 1 Fruit Exchange.

- - - - - - - - - -

Exchanges for one serving of the entire menu equal 1 Milk, 1 A Vegetable, 1 Fruit, 1 Bread, 2 Meat.

* * * * *

HOBO PARTY

A hobo party is planned for boys only. The invitations could read:

> Please come to my Hobo Party (it's only for boys, because everyone knows that girls never like to wear hobo clothes to a party).
>
> _____(signature)
>   Phone number: _____
> Date:_____Time: _____

To save time and money the child giving the party can deliver the invitations.

Menu and Recipes for Four

HOBO Special

Cold Drinks

HOBO Special

Clinkers*

Grape Icebergs

Cold Drinks (4 servings — 1 bottle or can each)

Provide four cans or bottles containing any desired flavor of sugar-free diet drinks, well chilled. Serve direct from containers or pour into paper cups in which ice cubes have been placed. *One serving equals Zero Exchange.*

Hobo Special (4 servings — 1 packet each)

　　12　*ounces lean ground Beef*
　　2　*medium-sized Carrots, sliced*
　　2　*medium-sized Potatoes, diced*
　　4　*thin slices of Onion*
　Salt and Pepper
　　4　*12-inch squares of heavy-duty Aluminum Foil*

Divide vegetables equally among the foil squares. Season and top with meat. Pull the four corners of foil together to form a pouch and twist to seal. Bake in 350-degree oven for 45 minutes.

*Contains small amount of sugar.

Place the packets in a pot or other container that has been suspended over the "campfire." Serve with spoons, allowing each boy to open his own packet.

One serving equals ½ B Vegetable Exchange, 1 Bread Exchange, 2 Meat Exchanges.

Clinkers (4 servings—1 each)

4   plain (unsugared) Cake Doughnuts*

Serve one doughnut to each boy.
One serving equals 1 Bread Exchange, 2 Fat Exchanges.

Grape Icebergs (4 servings—2 Icebergs each)

½   package Grape Kool-Aid, unsweetened
½   cup granulated Sucaryl
4   cups Water

Mix well, freeze, with sticks inserted, in frozen-sucker molds.
One serving equals Zero Exchange.

- - - - - - - - - -

Exchanges for one serving of the entire menu equal ½ B Vegetable, 2 Bread, 2 Meat, 2 Fat.

* * * * *

*Contains small amount of sugar.

BIRTHDAY PARTY

Come one, come all to the GREATEST SHOW ON
EARTH—with clowns and animals and lots of fun.
Games! Food! Cake! Ice Cream! Circus will be held
at ___ o'clock, on _____ , at the home of _____

This is a plan-ahead party for children from 6 to 10 years of
age. Invitations should be sent a week before the party, written
on animal cutouts. The exchange count should be given to the
mothers who will need this information.

Since eye appeal is important to children, the house or garden
may become a circus tent. In the house, crepe paper streamers
extending from the center of the ceiling to the four walls will give
a circus-tent effect. A real tent may be used in the garden. Provide many balloons and a special one for each child with his or
her name painted on it. Meet the children at the door dressed as
a clown. This will get the party off to a good start.

If the weather is cold or wet, ask each small guest to bring his
or her favorite stuffed animal. For a game, blindfold the children
and have them feel each other's animals and guess what they are.
Instead of the old game of "pin the tail on the donkey," have the
children pin a trunk on an elephant.

Instead of giving prizes to those who win games, present each
child with a gift. The gift can be an animal made of metal or
plastic, or, possibly, a coloring book of animal pictures.

Menu and Recipes for Four

Chicken Wing Drumsticks

Kool-Aid

Chicken Wing Drumsticks

Cherry Tomatoes

Birthday Cake with Frosting*

Ice Cream

Kool-Aid

1   package (any flavor) unsweetened Kool-Aid
1   cup granulated Sucaryl
2   quarts cold Water

Prepare Kool-Aid according to instructions on package using granulated Sucaryl instead of sugar. Serve over ice cubes.
One serving equals Zero Exchange.

Chicken Wing Drumsticks
(4 servings—4 little drumsticks each)

16   Chicken Wing Drumsticks
8   teaspoons Margarine
Salt

*Contains small amount of sugar.

Frozen chicken wing drumsticks are excellent if they are available. If not, the drumstick portion of chicken wings may be used.

Melt the margarine and brush it on the drumsticks—not more than 2 teaspoons to each four drumsticks. Sprinkle with flour and place on a flat baking sheet that has been sprayed with PAM. Cook in 350-degree oven for 1 hour. (This can be done ahead of time.) When ready to serve, place the drumsticks under the broiler and, watching very carefully, let them come to a golden brown.

One serving equals 2 Meat Exchanges, 2 Fat Exchanges.

Cherry Tomatoes (4 servings—3 tomatoes each)

12   Cherry Tomatoes

Wash the tomatoes and serve them whole.
One serving equals ¹/₂ A Vegetable Exchange.

Birthday Cake*
(4 servings—¹/₄ cake or 1 generous slice each)

6   tablespoons Cake Flour
¹/₈   teaspoon Salt
8   teaspoons Sugar
4   Egg Whites
¹/₃   teaspoon Cream of Tartar
¹/₂   teaspoon Vanilla Flavoring
¹/₄   teaspoon Almond Flavoring
1   teaspoon liquid Sucaryl

Sift flour, sugar, and salt together four times. Beat egg whites until frothy and add cream of tartar, beating until stiff. Add flavorings and Sucaryl. Fold dry ingredients into this mixture and pour into a small tube pan (about 8 inches in diameter) that has been sprayed with PAM. Bake in 325-degree oven for 45 minutes or until cake shrinks slightly from edge of pan. Remove from oven and turn upside down to cool.

*Contains small amount of sugar.

Frosting for Birthday Cake

    1   *Egg White*
    1   *package D-Zerta, strawberry flavor*
    1   *cup boiling Water*
    1   *tablespoon granulated Sucaryl*

Combine egg white, D-Zerta, and Sucaryl in small bowl and mix well. While beating with electric mixer, add boiling water and continue beating until mixture forms peaks. Spread on cooled cake and refrigerate until ready to use.

One serving (cake and frosting) equals 1 Bread Exchange.

Vanilla Ice Cream (4 servings — ¹/₂ cup each)

Use one-half the recipe for Ice Cream given in Part IV (see Index).

One serving equals ³/₄ Milk Exchange.

- - - - - - - - - -

Exchanges for one serving of the entire menu equal ³/₄ Milk, ¹/₂ A Vegetable, 1 Bread, 2 Meat, 2 Fat.

* * * * *

TEA PARTY

Your daughter may prefer to keep her tea party an all-girl affair. If so, her friends will love an invitation like this:

Please Bring Your Dolly
For Tea and Supper
At My House

_____(name)
Phone: _____
Date:_____Time:_____

However, if boys must be included, the invitation may be phrased: "Please Bring Your Favorite Stuffed Animal . . . ."

The menu for this party is designed to keep the guests on their diets but make them feel very special and in a party mood.

Menu and Recipes for Four

Tuna Triangles

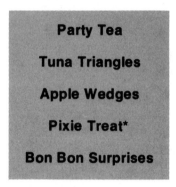

Party Tea

Tuna Triangles

Apple Wedges

Pixie Treat*

Bon Bon Surprises

Party Tea

Dilute 1 cup of tea with equal amount of water. Sweeten to taste with Sucaryl. Serve warm in doll tea pot. Put some milk in the creamer so that guests can help themselves to the "cream."
One serving equals Zero Exchange.

Tuna Triangles (4 servings—2 triangles each)

- 1/2   *cup water-packed Tuna Fish, minced*
- 4   *teaspoons Mayonnaise*
- 2   *slices Bread*
- 2   *tablespoons Milk*
- *Salt*

Mix tuna and mayonnaise, then add milk to moisten. Salt to taste. Spread the mixture on one of the bread slices and top with the other slice. Trim crusts very thin. Cut the sandwich into four squares; then cut each square into two triangles.
One serving equals 1/2 Bread Exchange, 1/2 Meat Exchange, 1 Fat Exchange.

*Contains small amount of sugar.

Apple Wedges (4 servings — ¹/₄ apple each)

1   *large Apple*
Lemon Juice

A fruit divider is useful for cutting the apple. If one is not available, core the whole apple, then cut it vertically into 12 thin wedges. Dip each wedge in lemon juice to prevent discoloration.
One serving equals ¹/₂ Fruit Exchange.

Pixie Treat* (4 servings — 1 sandwich each)

3   *tablespoons Cake Flour*
4   *teaspoons Sugar*
2   *Egg Whites*
¹/₆   *teaspoon Cream of Tartar*
¹/₆   *teaspoon Vanilla Flavoring*
¹/₈   *teaspoon Almond Flavoring*
¹/₂   *teaspoon liquid Sucaryl*
Pinch of Salt
1   *package D-Zerta (preferably red in color)*

Sift flour, salt, and sugar together several times. Beat egg whites until frothy; add cream of tartar and beat until stiff but not dry. Add flavorings and Sucaryl, and stir. Fold dry ingredients into egg whites.

Spray a cookie sheet with PAM. Use a pastry tube or a table-spoon and make eight finger-shaped mounds of the mixture. Bake in 325-degree oven for 15 to 20 minutes or until set and slightly brown. Let cool in pan, then remove gently with a spatula.

Dissolve one package of D-Zerta according to instructions on the container. Pour the solution into a flat pan so that it is not more than ¹/₄ inch in depth. When congealed, cut four portions, each the size of a cake finger. Put one layer of D-Zerta between two fingers of cake and press lightly so that cake and D-Zerta

*Contains small amount of sugar.

will stick together. Place each "sandwich" in the freezer for a few minutes before serving.

One serving equals ¹/₂ Bread Exchange.

Bon Bon Surprise
(4 servings—2 pieces candy and 3 peanuts each)

    8   *pieces wrapped hard Diabetic Candy*
   12   *shelled roasted Peanuts*

Each serving consists of two pieces of candy and three peanuts in a paper bon bon cup.

One serving equals Zero Exchange.

- - - - - - - - - -

Exchanges for one serving of the entire menu equal ¹/₂ Fruit, 1 Bread, ¹/₂ Meat, 1 Fat.

* * * * *

SEATED DINNERS

Every youngster loves to be invited to eat at the home of his or her "best friend." Usually, if there is only one guest, this child will be included at the family table, but if two or three children are invited, it will be more thrilling for them (and easier for you) if they sit by themselves.

A card table, covered with a bright plastic cloth, and paper plates and napkins may be used. The decor can be in the favorite color of the young host or hostess. At holiday times, hues characterizing the season are appropriate. Paper hats (made from folded newspaper or construction paper), balloons, and a centerpiece of flowers add to the party atmosphere.

Invitations for dinner may be given by phone by the child hosting the dinner, but the child's mother should check promptly with the guests' parents to make certain that they understand the date and hour. At this time the parent(s) of the diabetic guest(s) can be told what food exchanges will be served.

Menus and Recipes for Four

Spaghetti and Meat Sauce

Milk

Spaghetti and Meat Sauce

Celery and Carrot Strips

Melon Balls

Milk

Serve each child one 8-ounce glass of milk.
One glass equals 1 Milk Exchange.

Spaghetti and Meat Sauce (4 servings — 1 cup each)

1	cup cut Spaghetti
³/₄	pound lean ground Beef
2	ounces Tomato Paste
1¹/₂	teaspoons Salt
¹/₂	clove Garlic, crushed
¹/₂	teaspoon Oregano
¹/₈	teaspoon Sweet Basil
¹/₄	teaspoon Onion Powder
1	cup Water
1	Bay Leaf

Artificial sweetener to taste

Cook spaghetti according to directions on the package. Drain. Brown meat over medium heat in a large heavy skillet. Add tomato paste, stir, and cook with the meat for a few seconds. Add the cooked spaghetti and the remaining ingredients and mix well. Simmer for 2 hours. Add water if too thick.

One serving equals 1 Bread Exchange, 2 Meat Exchanges.

Celery and Carrot Strips (4 servings)

4   ribs Celery
2   Carrots

Scrub carrots and celery. Cut into small strips, about ¼ by 2 inches. Divide equally into four servings.

One serving equals ½ A Vegetable Exchange, ½ B Vegetable Exchange.

Melon Balls (4 servings—1 cup each)

1   medium-sized Cantaloupe or ½ small Watermelon

With a melon scoop, make enough melon balls to have 1 cup per serving.

One serving equals 1 Fruit Exchange.

- - - - - - - - - -

Exchanges for one serving of the entire menu equal 1 Milk, ½ A Vegetable, ½ B Vegetable, 1 Fruit, 1 Bread, 2 Meat.

* * * * *

Baked Turkey*

Milk

Baked Turkey

Mashed Potatoes   **Buttered Green Beans**

Pink Applesauce

Ice Cream Sandwich†

Milk

Serve each child one 8-ounce glass of milk.
One glass equals 1 Milk Exchange.

Baked Turkey (4 servings — 2 ounces each)

Use recipe for Holiday Turkey given in Part III (see Index).
One serving equals 2 Meat Exchanges.

---

*This menu can be used when turkey is left over from a previous meal. Chicken may be substituted for turkey.
†Contains small amount of sugar.

Mashed Potatoes (4 servings — ¹/₂ cup each)

> 2   medium-sized Potatoes, peeled
> ¹/₂ cup Milk
> 4   teaspoons Margarine
> Salt

Cook potatoes in small amount of salted water until tender (about ¹/₂ hour). Mash thoroughly. Add margarine, milk, and salt to taste; whip until fluffy. Serve hot.

One serving equals 1 Bread Exchange, 1 Fat Exchange.

Buttered Green Beans (4 servings — ¹/₄ cup each)

> ¹/₂ 16-ounce can cut Green Beans
> 2   teaspoons Margarine

Heat beans, in their own juice, to the boiling point. Drain, add margarine, and stir lightly.

One serving equals 1 A Vegetable Exchange, ¹/₂ Fat Exchange.

Pink Applesauce (4 servings — ¹/₂ cup each)

> 4   small, tart Apples
> ¹/₂   cup Water
> 1¹/₂ teaspoons liquid Sucaryl
> Red Cake Coloring

Peel, core, and slice apples. Add Sucaryl to water and pour over apples in a saucepan. Cover and cook slowly for 20 to 30 minutes, or until soft. Add food coloring as desired. Serve cold.

One serving equals 1 Fruit Exchange.

Ice Cream Sandwich*
(4 servings — 1 ice cream sandwich each)

3	tablespoons Cake Flour
4	teaspoons Sugar
2	Egg Whites

Pinch of Salt

$1/6$	teaspoon Cream of Tartar
$1/6$	teaspoon Vanilla Flavoring
$1/8$	teaspoon Almond Flavoring
$1/2$	teaspoon liquid Sucaryl
4	tablespoons Cool Whip

Sift flour, salt, and sugar together several times. Beat egg whites until frothy, add cream of tartar, beat until stiff but not dry. Add flavorings and Sucaryl and stir. Fold dry ingredients into egg whites quickly.

Shape into eight oval patties on a cookie sheet that has been sprayed with PAM. Bake in 325-degree oven for 15 to 20 minutes, or until brown. Cool thoroughly. Make sandwiches of two patties and 1 tablespoon Cool Whip each. Put in freezer until ready to serve.

One serving equals $1/2$ Bread Exchange.

- - - - - - - - - -

Exchanges for one serving of the entire menu equal 1 Milk, 1 A Vegetable, 1 Fruit, 1½ Bread, 2 Meat, 1½ Fat.

* * * * *

*Contains small amount of sugar.

Broiled Fish

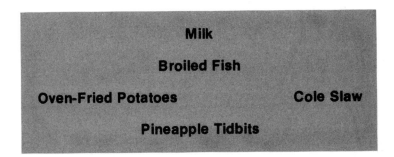

Milk

Broiled Fish

Oven-Fried Potatoes   **Cole Slaw**

Pineapple Tidbits

Milk

Serve each child one 8-ounce glass of milk.
One glass equals 1 Milk Exchange.

Broiled Fish (4 servings—2 ounces each)

> 12 ounces thin *Fish Fillets, uncooked*
> 4   teaspoons *Cooking Oil*
> *Salt and Pepper*

Place fillets in shallow broiling pan that has been sprayed with PAM. Brush 2 teaspoons of oil over top of fish. Broil in oven until top is brown. Turn over and brush the rest of oil on fish. Return to broiler until top is brown. Divide into four portions; serve hot.
One serving equals 2 Meat Exchanges, 1 Fat Exchange.

Oven-Fried Potatoes (4 servings—¹/₂ potato each)

> 2 medium-sized *Potatoes*
> 4 teaspoons *Cooking Oil*
> *Seasoned Salt*

Scrub unpeeled potatoes with brush and cut into slices about
$1/3$ inch thick. Place slices on broiler pan that has been sprayed
with PAM; sprinkle with salt, and rub with half the oil. Bake in
400-degree oven for about 10 minutes or until brown. Remove
from oven, turn potato slices over, and rub on the rest of the oil.
Return potatoes to oven; remove when brown.
   One serving equals 1 Bread Exchange, 1 Fat Exchange.

Cole Slaw (4 servings — $1/2$ cup each)

   $1/4$ medium-sized Cabbage, chopped
   6   tablespoons Evaporated Milk
   4   teaspoons Vinegar
   $1/3$ teaspoon Celery Seed
   $1/2$ teaspoon liquid Sucaryl
   Pinch of Salt

   Mix milk, vinegar, celery seed, salt, and liquid Sucaryl. Pour
over chopped cabbage and stir.
   One serving equals 1 A Vegetable Exchange.

Pineapple Tidbits (4 servings — $1/2$ cup each)

   1   can (about 16 ounces) unsweetened Pineapple Tid-
       bits, chilled

Serve very cold.
One serving equals 1 Fruit Exchange.

- - - - - - - - - -

   *Exchanges for one serving of the entire menu equal 1 Milk, 1
A Vegetable, 1 Fruit, 1 Bread, 2 Meat, 2 Fat.*

* * * * *

Barbecued Beefies

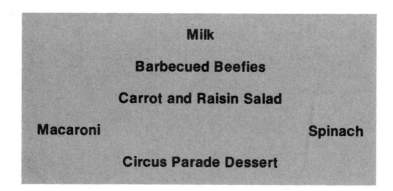

Milk

Barbecued Beefies

Carrot and Raisin Salad

Macaroni   **Spinach**

Circus Parade Dessert

Milk

Serve each child one 8-ounce glass of milk.
One glass equals 1 Milk Exchange.

Barbecued Beefies (4 servings — 1 Beefy each)

12	*ounces lean ground Beef*
1	*Egg*
1	*slice Bread, crumbled*
$^1/_2$	*cup Skim Milk*
$^1/_2$	*teaspoon Salt*
$^1/_4$	*teaspoon Pepper*
$^1/_2$	*teaspoon Celery Salt*

Beat egg and milk together; add bread crumbs and seasoning. Mix well and add meat. Shape into four small loaves. Place in casserole that has been sprayed with PAM. Bake in 350-degree oven for 1¹/₄ hours, basting occasionally with Barbecue Sauce (recipe follows).

For plain meat loaf, barbecue sauce may be omitted.

Barbecue Sauce (4 servings—3 tablespoons each)

3   ounces *Tomato Paste*
³/₄   cup hot *Water*
1¹/₂   tablespoons *Vinegar*
¹/₄   teaspoon liquid *Sucaryl*
¹/₂   teaspoon *Salt*
1   tablespoon *Worcestershire Sauce*

Mix water and tomato paste in saucepan. Add remaining ingredients; simmer for about 1 hour.

One serving of barbecued beefies equals 2 Meat Exchanges.

Carrot and Raisin Salad (4 servings — ¹/₄ cup each)

1   cup coarsely grated *Carrot*
2   tablespoons *Raisins*
8   teaspoons *Mayonnaise*
1   tablespoon *Milk*
¹/₄   teaspoon liquid *Sucaryl*
¹/₄   teaspoon *Salt*

Pour boiling water over raisins to plump them. Drain well. Combine all ingredients. Serve cold on lettuce leaf.

One serving equals ¹/₂ B Vegetable Exchange, 2 Fat Exchanges.

Macaroni (4 servings — ¹/₂ cup each)

1   cup *Macaroni, broken in bits*
¹/₂   teaspoon *Butter Flavoring*
¹/₂   teaspoon *Salt*

Boil macaroni in salted water according to instructions given on package. Drain well, reserving 1 tablespoon of the water. Combine water and flavoring, and pour over cooked macaroni. Serve hot.

One serving equals 1 Bread Exchange.

Spinach (4 servings — 1/4 cup each)

1   *package frozen Spinach (about 10 ounces)*
1/2   *teaspoon Salt*
1/2   *teaspoon Butter Flavoring or 1 tablespoon Vinegar*

Cook spinach according to directions on package. Drain. Add butter flavoring or vinegar. If vinegar is used, sprinkle a bit of pepper over the top of the spinach.
One serving equals 1/2 A Vegetable Exchange.

Circus Parade Dessert (4 servings — 1 "parade" each)

4   *Graham Cracker squares*
4   *tablespoons Peanut Butter*
12   *Animal Crackers*

Spread 1 tablespoon peanut butter on each graham cracker. Stand three animal crackers on each graham cracker.
One serving equals 1 Bread Exchange, 1/2 Meat Exchange.

- - - - - - - - - -

Exchanges for one serving of the entire menu equal 1 Milk, 1/2 A Vegetable, 1/2 B Vegetable, 2 Bread, 2 1/2 Meat, 2 Fat.

* * * * *

Broiled Steak

Milk

Steak

Mashed Potatoes

Buttered Peas   **Carrot Sticks**

Strawberry Sundae

Milk

Serve each child one 8-ounce glass of milk.
One glass equals 1 Milk Exchange.

Broiled Steak (4 servings—2 ounces each)

12   *ounces tender broiling Steak*
Salt and Pepper

Broil steak until it is rare, medium, or well-done as desired.
One serving equals 2 Meat Exchanges.

Mashed Potatoes (4 servings—¹/₂ cup each)

2   *medium-sized Potatoes*
3   *tablespoons Evaporated Milk*
¹/₂   *teaspoon Butter Flavoring*
Salt

Peel potatoes and boil them in a small amount of salted water in a saucepan until done (about ¹/₂ hour). Put potatoes in mixer bowl, saving the water in which they were boiled. Add butter flavoring to milk and pour over potatoes. Beat with mixer until fluffy. If necessary, add some of the water in which potatoes were boiled to obtain the right consistency.

One serving equals 1 Bread Exchange.

Buttered Peas (4 servings — ¹/₂ cup each)

1	package (10 ounces) frozen Green Peas
4	teaspoons Margarine
¹/₂	teaspoon Salt

Cook peas according to directions on package. Drain and add margarine.

One serving equals 1 B Vegetable Exchange, 1 Fat Exchange.

Carrot Sticks (4 servings — several sticks each)

3	raw Carrots

Scrub carrots with brush while washing them. (Scraping is not necessary, but it may be done if preferred.) Cut carrots lengthwise into strips about ¹/₄ inch wide, then cut into 2- or 3-inch lengths.

One serving equals ¹/₂ B Vegetable Exchange.

Strawberry Sundae

Vanilla Ice Cream (4 servings — ¹/₂ cup each)

For ice cream use recipe given in Part IV (see Index). Because this recipe is for eight servings of ¹/₂ cup each, one half of it should be used here.

Strawberry Topping (4 servings — ¼ cup each)

1   *cup unsweetened sliced Strawberries*

Serve the strawberries over the top of each dish of ice cream. *One serving of the sundae equals* ¾ *Milk Exchange,* ¼ *Fruit Exchange.*

- - - - - - - - - -

Exchanges for one serving of the entire menu equal 1¾ *Milk,* 1½ *B Vegetable,* ¼ *Fruit, 1 Bread, 2 Meat, 1 Fat.*

* * * * *

PART II

Parties for the Diabetic

Teenager

or

Young Adult

COOKOUTS

Cookouts have special appeal for teenagers and young adults as they provide the stage for action. If you have no backyard facilities for such a party, don't fret. The group may be taken to the nearest park. In backyard or park, let the guests cook their own meat, but make certain that they are given the proper portions.

Invite someone who has a guitar, accordion, or other musical instrument, and soon the whole group will be singing.

Hopefully the weather will be fine, but if it rains and the party cannot be postponed there are alternatives to the out-of-doors. If you have no porch or recreation room, the living room will do nicely. The guest may be seated on the living room floor, but 'twill be best if only one or two cooks hold forth in the kitchen.

In the winter, a "snow barbecue" will be enjoyed, that is, if you live in a section of the country in which the "white stuff" falls. Ask guests to dress warmly. They will enjoy making a snowman or two, even engaging in snowball battles just like "when they were kids."

Menus and Recipes for Eight

Barbecued Chicken

Iced Tea

Potato Salad

Barbecued Chicken   **Assorted Diced Fruits**

Chocolate Ice Cream Sundae

Potato Salad (8 servings—1¹/₄ cups each)

8	cups boiled Potatoes, diced
6	tablespoons Mayonnaise
8	Eggs, hard-boiled and chopped
1	cup Evaporated Milk
¹/₂	cup Vinegar
¹/₂	cup minced Onion
1	tablespoon Prepared Mustard
2	Green Peppers, minced
6	Dill Pickles, chopped
2	teaspoons Celery Seed
Salt	

Add vinegar, celery seed, and mayonnaise to the diced potatoes, and stir. Add remaining ingredients. Let stand for 1 hour or more so that the potatoes will absorb the salt and vinegar seasonings. Taste, and add more salt if desired. Refrigerate and serve cold.

One serving equals 2 Bread Exchanges, 1 A Vegetable Exchange, 1 Meat Exchange, 2 Fat Exchanges.

Barbecued Chicken (8 servings — ¹/₄ chicken each)

> 2 *3-pound frying Chickens*
> 1¹/₂ *cups Barbecue Sauce (recipe follows)*
> *Salt and Pepper*

Wash and quarter chickens; dry with paper towels. Rub on salt and pepper. Prepare a bed of coals using charcoal, or, if you have a gas grill, let the coals heat for several minutes. Place chickens on grill, not too close to coals. Watch carefully and turn frequently. When chickens are about half done, brush with barbecue sauce; then each time they are turned brush with more sauce. Cook until golden brown (a total of 1 to 1¹/₄ hours).

Barbecue Sauce

> 1 *can (6 ounces) Tomato Paste*
> 1¹/₂ *cups hot Water*
> 3 *tablespoons Vinegar*
> ¹/₂ *teaspoon liquid Sucaryl*
> ¹/₄ *teaspoon Chili Powder*
> ¹/₂ *teaspoon Garlic Salt*
> 1 *teaspoon Salt*
> 1 *pinch Cayenne Pepper*
> 3 *tablespoons Worcestershire Sauce*
> ¹/₂ *teaspoon Liquid Smoke*
> 1 *teaspoon minced dried Onions*
> 3 *tablespoons Salad Oil*

Mix water and tomato paste in a saucepan. Add remaining ingredients. Salt to taste. Simmer for 1 hour. This will yield about 1¹/₂ cups of sauce that will be quite thick.

One serving of barbecued chicken equals 3 Meat Exchanges, 1 Fat Exchange.

Assorted Fruits (8 servings — 2 fruit exchanges each)

From available fresh fruits, choose enough to make up 16 Fruit Exchanges. Divide into portions so that guests can serve themselves (2 Fruit Exchanges each).

Chocolate Ice Cream Sundae

Vanilla Ice Cream (8 servings — 1/2 cup each)

Use recipe given for Ice Cream in Part IV (see Index).

Chocolate Syrup (8 servings — 2 1/2 tablespoons each)

    1 1/2   cups *Evaporated Milk*
    1/2   cup *unsweetened Cocoa*
    1/4   teaspoon *Salt*
    1 1/2   teaspoons *liquid Sucaryl*
    1   teaspoon *Vanilla Flavoring*

Combine cocoa with 4 tablespoons of the evaporated milk; mix until smooth. Add salt and remaining milk slowly while stirring. Cook over very low heat until mixture is smooth. Remove from heat, add vanilla flavoring; cool, add Sucaryl, and mix thoroughly. When ready to serve, pour over ice cream in individual portions.

One serving of ice cream and chocolate syrup equals 1 1/4 Milk Exchanges.

- - - - - - - - - -

Exchanges for one serving of the entire menu equal 1 1/4 Milk, 1 A Vegetable, 2 Fruit, 2 Bread, 4 Meat, 3 Fat.

* * * * *

Weiners and Cheese on Buns

Weiners and Cheese on Buns

Tomato Wedges with Celery and Carrot Sticks

Dill Pickles

Banana Milk Shake

Weiners and Cheese on Buns
(8 servings—2 weiners, 2 strips of cheese, 2 buns each)

16   *Weiners (8 per pound)*
$1/2$ *pound sharp Cheddar Cheese*
16   *Hot Dog Buns*
Jar of Prepared Mustard

Cut cheese into 16 equal strips. Cook weiners, on long roasting forks or on sharpened sticks, over hot coals. Buns may also be toasted over the fire if desired. Slit buns lengthwise and insert one strip of cheese and one weiner in each.
One serving equals 2 Bread Exchanges, 3 Meat Exchanges.

Tomato Wedges with Celery and Carrot Sticks (8 servings)

4   *medium-sized Tomatoes*
4   *ribs Celery*
8   *small Carrots*
8   *Dill Pickles*

Cut tomatoes in quarters; cut celery and carrots into strips; serve dill pickles whole or sliced.
One serving equals 1 A Vegetable Exchange, $1/2$ B Vegetable Exchange.

Banana Milk Shake (8 servings — 1¹/₄ cups each)'

8	small Bananas
8	cups whole Milk
1	cup Orange Juice
¹/₄	teaspoon Salt
4	teaspoons liquid Sucaryl
¹/₂	teaspoon Almond Flavoring

Combine all ingredients in blender and blend until frothy. Serve very cold in parfait or other tall glasses.

One serving equals 1 Milk Exchange, 2¹/₄ Fruit Exchanges.

- - - - - - - - - -

Exchanges for one serving of the entire menu equal 1 Milk, 1 A Vegetable, ¹/₂ B Vegetable, 2¹/₄ Fruit, 2 Bread, 3 Meat.

* * * * *

Grilled Hamburgers

Grilled Hamburgers with Onion, Mustard, Pickle, and Lettuce

Celery and Carrot Strips

Frozen Ice Cream Sandwiches

Assorted Diet Drinks

Grilled Hamburgers (8 servings—2 patties each)

3   *pounds lean ground Beef*
16   *small Buns*
2   *Onions, sliced thin*
Prepared Mustard
2   *Dill Pickles, sliced thin*
Lettuce leaves
Salt and Pepper

Mix meat with salt and pepper and shape into 16 patties, 3 ounces each. Split buns in half, wrap in aluminum foil, and place on back of grill to keep warm. Cook meat patties over hot coals, place in hot buns. Serve two per person.

Condiment suggestion for hamburgers: Spread out 16 lettuce leaves, put onion and pickle slices on each leaf. Keep refrigerated until ready to use.

One serving (2 hamburgers plus pickles, onions, and lettuce) equals 2 Bread Exchanges, 4 Meat Exchanges.

Celery and Carrot Strips
(8 servings — ¹/₂ carrot and 1 strip of celery each)

Prepare vegetables for eating with fingers. Keep cold in plastic bag until ready to serve.

One serving equals ¹/₂ A Vegetable Exchange, ¹/₂ B Vegetable Exchange.

Frozen Ice Cream Sandwiches
(8 servings — 2 sandwiches with topping each)

1¹/₂	cups powdered Skim Milk
8	teaspoons liquid Sucaryl
1	teaspoon Vanilla Flavoring
12	Egg Whites
4	cups Jane's topping*

Beat egg whites until they will stand in peaks. Add Sucaryl and vanilla flavoring. Add powdered milk slowly, beating constantly until the mixture is the consistency of a smooth paste. Spoon finger-shaped cakes about 2 inches wide and 4 inches long onto a cookie sheet that has been sprayed with PAM. Do not let the cakes touch each other. This recipe will make 32 cakes. Bake in 275-degree oven for 40 minutes. Remove carefully from pan. When cool put ¹/₄ cup of Jane's topping between 2 cakes. Freeze until ready to serve.

One serving (two sandwiches with topping) equals 1 Skim Milk Exchange. (¹/₄ cup of topping alone equals Zero Exchange.)

- - - - - - - - - -

Exchanges for one serving of the entire menu equal 1 Skim Milk, ¹/₂ A Vegetable, ¹/₂ B Vegetable, 2 Bread, 4 Meat.

* * * * *

*Double the recipe for Jane's topping given in Part IV (see Index).

Chili—Cowboy Style

Diet Bottled Drinks

Chili—Cowboy Style

Assorted Fruits in Season

Lemon Snaps*

Chili—Cowboy Style (8 servings — ³/₄ cup each)

2	pounds lean ground Beef
4	large Onions, chopped
3	tablespoons Chili Powder
2	cans Tomatoes (about 1 pound each)
1	teaspoon Oregano
2	cloves Garlic, crushed
2	teaspoons Salt
1	teaspoon Cumin Seed
2	cups Hot Water
8	corn Tortillas (5 or 6 inches in diameter)
8	ounces American Cheese, grated
4	cups fresh Tomatoes, chopped

Put meat, garlic, and onions in a large heavy skillet and sear until lightly browned. Add chili powder, oregano, canned tomatoes, salt, cumin, and hot water. Bring to a boil, then lower heat and simmer for 2 hours. Let set until cold and skim off fat. Before reheating, measure volume; if necessary add water to make 6 cups.

*Contain small amount of sugar.

Place tortillas on cookie sheet and salt slightly. Bake in 325-degree oven for 30 minutes, or until lightly browned and crisp.

Serve in deep pottery bowls or cereal bowls. Each guest takes a toasted tortilla, breaks it into bite-size pieces, and puts them in a bowl. Add ³/₄ cup of hot chili mixture on top of tortilla pieces, then add a generous portion of chopped fresh tomato over chili. Top with 2 tablespoons of grated cheese. Serve with soup spoons.

One serving equals 1 A Vegetable Exchange, ¹/₂ B Vegetable Exchange, 1 Bread Exchange, 4 Meat Exchanges.

Assorted Fruits in Season

Conforming to the Exchange System, use available fruits in season. Allow 2 Fruit Exchanges per guest.

Lemon Snaps*

Serve 6 small lemon snaps to each person.
One serving (6 cookies) equals 1 Bread Exchange.

- - - - - - - - - -

Exchanges for one serving of the entire menu equal 1 A Vegetable, ¹/₂ B Vegetable, 2 Fruit, 2 Bread, 4 Meat.

* * * * *

*Contain small amount of sugar.

Broiled Steak

Hot Bean-Bacon Soup

Broiled Steak

Buttered French Bread

Cole Slaw

Watermelon and Cantaloupe

Bean-Bacon Soup (8 servings — 1 cup each)

Prepare four cans of condensed Bean-with-Bacon Soup according to directions on can. Serve hot in mugs.

One serving equals 1½ Bread Exchanges, 1 Meat Exchange.

Broiled Steak (8 servings — 3 ounces cooked meat each)

    2   pounds Eye-of-the-Round Steak*
    8   teaspoons Margarine
    1   teaspoon Lemon Juice
    Salt and Pepper

Sprinkle the slices of steak with salt and pepper. Melt margarine and add lemon juice. Prepare a bed of coals in the grill. Brush both sides of each steak with the margarine mixture. Broil the steaks over the hot coals for a minute or so on each side. Serve hot.

One serving equals 3 Meat Exchanges, 1 Fat Exchange.

*Have your butcher cut the steak into eight slices and run the slices through the tenderizer.

Buttered French Bread (8 servings—2 slices each)

   1   *one-pound loaf French Bread*
  16   *teaspoons Margarine*
  Garlic Salt

Cut bread, almost through, into 16 equal slices. Spread each slice with 1 teaspoon margarine that has been warmed to room temperature. Shake garlic salt between slices of bread. Roll the bread in foil and place on back of grill so that it can be served hot.

One serving equals 2 Bread Exchanges, 2 Fat Exchanges.

Cole Slaw (8 servings—1 cup each)

   1   *firm 3-pound head of Cabbage (to yield 8 cups when chopped)*
  1½   *cups canned Skim Milk*
  ½   *cup Vinegar*
   2   *teaspoons liquid Sucaryl*
   2   *tablespoons Celery Seed*
   1   *teaspoon Salt*

Trim cabbage and chop fine. Mix the other ingredients. When ready to serve, pour the mixture over the cabbage and toss thoroughly. (If slaw is allowed to stand too long, dressing will separate.)

One serving equals ¼ Milk Exchange, 1 A Vegetable Exchange.

Watermelon and Cantaloupe
(8 servings—1 piece of each fruit for each serving)

   8   *slices Watermelon (3 by 3 by 1½ inches)*
   2   *6-inch Cantaloupes, cut in quarters*

One serving *(of melon and cantaloupe) equals 2 Fruit Exchanges.*

- - - - - - - - - -

Exchanges for one serving of the entire menu equal ¹/₄ Milk, 1 A Vegetable, 2 Fruit, 3¹/₂ Bread, 4 Meat, 3 Fat.

* * * * *

SWIM PARTY

Be grateful that the "Ole Swimmin' Hole" isn't what it used to be. Today you can send or take your teenagers for a swim and fun in countless places where lifeguards are in attendance. Somewhere close to you there probably will be clean, clear fresh-water ponds or lakes, ocean beaches, or public or private swimming pools.

Take advantage of enthusiasm for water sports and plan a swimming party and box lunch for your son or daughter. Such a party provides a wonderful way to entertain visiting cousins or friends.

After the young people have worn themselves out in the water they will be starved and will be delighted to be given a box lunch filled with goodies. Add a personal note by painting names on the boxes in bold letters.

Menu and Recipes for Six

Fried Chicken-Tuna Sandwiches

Assorted Diet Drinks

Iced Tea

Fried Chicken   **Tuna Sandwiches**

Boiled Eggs

Bread Sticks

Raw Vegetables   **Green Onion Dip**

Fresh Fruit

Take-alongs: Salt and Pepper Packets, Sugar-Substitute Packets (for the iced tea), Paper Napkins, Paper Cups, Wash-and-Dry Towelettes, Ice.

Fried Chicken (6 servings—2 pieces chicken each)

6   *Chicken Drumsticks*
6   *Chicken Thighs*
1   *tablespoon Cooking Oil*
Salt and Pepper
Paprika

Spray cookie sheet with PAM. Brush chicken pieces with oil. Sprinkle with paprika, salt, and pepper; place on cookie sheet. Bake in 400-degree oven for 20 minutes. Turn chicken pieces and bake another 25 minutes.

One serving (2 pieces of chicken) equals 2 Meat Exchanges, 1 Fat Exchange.

Tuna Sandwiches (6 servings — 1 sandwich each)

> 2   cans (6½ ounces each) water-packed Tuna Fish
> 4   tablespoons Mayonnaise
> 4   tablespoons grated Onion
> ½   cup Celery, finely minced
> Bread

Drain tuna fish. Mix all ingredients until smooth. Use two thin slices (about 30 slices per 1-pound loaf) of bread and ¼ cup of tuna mixture for each sandwich. Cut each sandwich into triangles and place in a sandwich bag and keep in the refrigerator until you are ready to assemble the boxes.

One serving (one whole sandwich) equals 1½ Bread Exchanges, 2 Meat Exchanges, 2 Fat Exchanges.

Boiled Eggs

Hard-boil 6 eggs. Do not peel. Put one egg with salt and pepper packets in each box.

One serving (1 egg) equals 1 Meat Exchange.

Bread Sticks (6 servings — two 9-inch sticks each)

One serving equals ½ Bread Exchange.

Raw Vegetables (6 servings — assorted vegetables)

> 6   medium-sized Carrots
> 6   ribs Celery
> 18   Radishes
> 18   Cherry Tomatoes

Prepare vegetables for dipping. Other vegetables, such as cauliflower and green pepper strips, can be added if desired.

One serving of assorted vegetables equals 1 A Vegetable Exchange, 1 B Vegetable Exchange.

Green Onion Dip (6 servings — ¹/₄ cup each)

1	cup *Sour Cream*
¹/₂	cup *Buttermilk*
1	tablespoon *Water*
1	package *Green Onion Dip mix*
¹/₂	teaspoon *Gelatin*
¹/₄	teaspoon *Salt*

Sprinkle gelatin on water. When clear, heat until dissolved. Beat into buttermilk with hand mixer; blend in remaining ingredients.

One serving equals 1 Fat Exchange.

Fresh Fruit (6 servings — one fruit per person)

One small apple, orange, pear, or tangerine constitutes a serving.

One serving equals 1 Fruit Exchange.

- - - - - - - - - -

Exchanges for one serving of entire menu equal 1 A Vegetable, 1 B Vegetable, 1 Fruit, 2 Bread, 5 Meat, 4 Fat.

* * * * *

BUFFETS

Valentine Buffet

Hearts and flowers won't appeal to the boys until they become interested in girls. Then they will be delighted to be invited to a Valentine buffet supper and dance or party. Girls, of course, from the age 12 up, will love such a party.

Invitations can be written on valentines and valentines can be used for place cards. If the guests are brought to the party by their parents, rather than coming with their 'dates,' let them pick their dinner partners by matching red hearts cut into two odd sections. They will have fun coordinating the pieces.

Provide plenty of dance records. Your son or daughter will know which ones to get. If you have a non-dancing group, cards, charades, pinball, pool, or guessing games may be played.

Menu and Recipes for Ten

Barbecued Beefies

Diet Bottled Drinks

Barbecued Beefies

Green Peas   **Tomato Aspic**

Celery Sticks

Buttered French Bread

Valentine Pears

Barbecued Beefies (10 servings — one 3-ounce Beefy each)

2¹/₂ pounds lean Ground Beef
2   Eggs, beaten
1¹/₂ cups Milk
1¹/₂ cups soft Bread Crumbs
2   teaspoons Salt
¹/₂ teaspoon Pepper
1   teaspoon Worcestershire Sauce
2   teaspoons Celery Salt

Mix all ingredients and shape into 10 individual meat loaves. Place in greased casserole or pan. Pour half of the Sauce (recipe follows) over the top of the loaves. Bake in 350-degree oven for 1¹/₄ hours, basting occasionally with the remaining sauce.

Sauce for Beefies

4   *tablespoons Tomato Paste*
³/₄   *cup Water*
2   *tablespoons Vinegar*
¹/₂   *teaspoon liquid Sucaryl*
¹/₄   *teaspoon Chili Powder (more if desired)*
3   *teaspoons Salt*
1   *teaspoon Tabasco Sauce*

Mix the ingredients thoroughly.

One serving (beefy with sauce) equals ¹/₂ Bread Exchange, 3 Meat Exchanges, ¹/₂ Fat Exchange.

Green Peas (10 servings — ¹/₂ cup each)

3   *cans (about 17 ounces each) small Green Peas*
1   *teaspoon Butter Flavoring*

Drain most of the liquid from the peas, then stir in the butter flavoring and simmer for about 10 minutes. Serve hot.

One serving equals 1 B Vegetable Exchange.

Tomato Aspic (10 servings — ¹/₂ cup each)

5   *cups V-8 Cocktail Vegetable Juice*
5   *tablespoons Gelatin*
3   *tablespoons Mayonnaise*
1   *Beef Bouillon Cube*
¹/₂   *cup finely chopped Green Olives*

Sprinkle gelatin on 1 cup of cold V-8 Cocktail Vegetable Juice. Heat remainder of juice to boiling, then add bouillon cube. While still hot, add gelatin mixture and stir. Allow to cool and add chopped olives. Pour into individual heart molds, ¹/₂ cup each, and chill in refrigerator. Serve on lettuce. (Alternatively the whole mixture may be poured into a large heart mold, then served on a platter with lettuce.) Serve with mayonnaise, allowing 1 teaspoon per person.

One serving (aspic and mayonnaise) equals 1 A Vegetable Exchange, 1 Fat Exchange.

Celery Sticks (10 servings)

Prepare 10 ribs of celery, cut into small sticks.
One serving equals ½ A Vegetable Exchange.

Buttered French Bread (10 servings — 1 slice each)

1   *loaf French Bread (about 1 pound)*
10   *teaspoons Margarine*

Cut bread into slices about ¾ inch thick. On each of 10 slices spread 1 teaspoon margarine. Assemble slices into loaf-shape and wrap in aluminum foil. Heat in 325-degree oven for 20 minutes. Serve hot.

One serving equals 1 Bread Exchange, 1 Fat Exchange.

Valentine Pears (10 servings — 2 pear halves per serving)

20   *Pear halves, water packed*
3   *sticks Cinnamon*
Sucaryl to taste
Red Food Coloring

Dissolve the food coloring in the pear liquid until desired shade is achieved. Add Sucaryl and cinnamon sticks and simmer pears in liquid for 10 minutes, then remove cinnamon. Serve two pear halves with juice for each guest, in white or glass dessert dishes.

One serving equals 2 Fruit Exchanges.

- - - - - - - - - -

Exchanges for one serving of the entire menu equal 1½ A Vegetable, 1 B Vegetable, 2 Fruit, 1½ Bread, 3 Meat, 2½ Fat.

* * * * *

Hallowe'en Buffet

WITCHES, GHOSTS, AND GOBLINS WILL
GATHER FOR A COSTUME PARTY AND SUP-
PER ON HALLOWE'EN AT THE _____ .
*Brooms, Bags of Tricks, and Rattling Chains Must
Be Parked at the Door.*

Steaming brew served from a cauldron by a witch in costume
near the door will set the stage for an exciting evening. This party runs on its own momentum, for the masks, the costumes, and
the date make any gathering a gala affair.

Ideas for entertainment after supper include: (1) eating apples
suspended from rafter or ceiling on a string; (2) having the group
sit in a ring on the floor and announcing that a wicked werewolf
has just been killed, each person then adding one or two sen-
tences to the story behind the news—how the feat was ac-
complished, what happened to the witnesses, etc.; and (3) the
traditional telling of ghost stories.

Menu and Recipes for Ten

Ham Loaf

Witches' Brew

Ham Loaf

Scalloped Potatoes   **Cream Style Corn**

Golden Glow Salad

Bavarian Cream with Orange Sauce

Witches' Brew (10 servings — 12 ounces each)

10 cans *Apple-flavored Diet Drink*
2   sticks *Cinnamon*
3   whole *Cloves*

Heat the diet drink and add spices. Allow to steep, then remove spices. Serve warm in heat-proof paper cups. There will be enough for seconds.

One serving equals Zero Exchange.

Ham Loaf (10 servings — one loaf each)

1¹⁄₂ pounds cooked *Ham, ground*
¹⁄₂   cup *Cracker Crumbs*
1   cup *canned Skim Milk*
2   *Eggs*
1   teaspoon *Pepper*
¹⁄₄   teaspoon *Thyme*
1   cup *minced Onion*

Beat eggs slightly. Combine eggs with all other ingredients and mix well. Shape into 10 individual loaves. Bake in 350-degree oven for 20 minutes. Drizzle sauce (recipe follows) over ham loaves, then put them under broiler for 2 minutes.

Sauce for Ham Loaf (10 servings)

²/₃	cup Brown-Sugar Substitute
2	tablespoons Vinegar
1	teaspoon Dry Mustard
3	tablespoons Flour

Combine all ingredients and boil for 1 minute.
One serving (ham loaf with sauce) equals ¹/₂ Fruit Exchange, 3 Meat Exchanges.

Scalloped Potatoes (10 servings — 1 cup each)

7	medium-sized Potatoes
3	tablespoons Margarine
1	tablespoon Salt
3	tablespoons Flour
1	large Onion, minced
3	cups Milk
10	ounces Sharp Cheese, grated
	Pepper to taste
	Paprika

Boil potatoes, allow them to cool, then cut them into thin slices, and place in a casserole that has been sprayed with PAM. Sauté onions in the margarine, then after adding flour, salt, and pepper, stir in the milk. Cook this mixture until it thickens, then add the cheese to it and pour it over the potatoes. Bake in 325-degree oven for 40 minutes, or until slightly browned.
One serving equals ¹/₄ Milk Exchange, 2 Bread Exchanges, 1 Meat Exchange, 1 Fat Exchange.

Cream Style Corn (10 servings — ²/₃ cup each)

7 cups canned Cream Style Corn
10 teaspoons Margarine
Salt and Pepper

Mix all ingredients and heat to boiling point.
One serving equals 2 Bread Exchanges, 1 Fat Exchange.

Golden Glow Salad (10 servings — ¹/₂ cup each)

2 packages Orange-Flavored D-Zerta
2 cups boiling Water
2 cups unsweetened Pineapple Juice
2 cups unsweetened Pineapple, diced
2 cups Carrots, finely ground
2 teaspoons Salt
2 tablespoons Vinegar

Dissolve D-Zerta in hot water, add pineapple juice, salt, and vinegar. When mixture begins to thicken, add other ingredients and pour into individual molds to congeal. Serve on crisp greens.
One serving equals ¹/₂ B Vegetable Exchange, 1 Fruit Exchange.

Bavarian Cream with Orange Sauce
(10 servings — ¹/₂ cup each)

3 tablespoons Gelatin
³/₄ cup Water
6 Eggs, separated
3 cups Milk
Rind of 1 Orange, finely grated
³/₄ teaspoon Salt
³/₄ teaspoon liquid Sucaryl
3 teaspoons Vanilla Flavoring

Soak gelatin in cold water. Beat egg yolks, add salt and milk, then cook until mixture will coat a spoon. Add soaked gelatin and stir until gelatin is dissolved. Add Sucaryl and vanilla flavoring. Fold in stiffly beaten egg whites and grated orange rind. Pour into molds and chill in refrigerator. Serve with orange sauce (recipe follows).

Orange Sauce (10 servings—2 tablespoons each)

1	tablespoon Cornstarch
2	tablespoons cold Water
1	cup boiling Water
2	teaspoons Margarine
3	tablespoons Lemon Juice
2	teaspoons liquid Sucaryl
1	small pinch of Salt
2	medium-sized Oranges

Blend cornstarch and cold water. Add boiling water and boil mixture for 5 minutes, stirring constantly. Remove from fire and add margarine, lemon juice, Sucaryl, and salt. While this mixture is cooling, grate the rind from the oranges and cut the orange sections into small pieces. Add rind and orange sections to the mixture together with a little additional orange food coloring, if desired. Serve 2 tablespoons over each helping of Bavarian cream.

One serving (Bavarian cream with sauce) equals ¼ Milk Exchange, 1 Fruit Exchange, 1 Meat Exchange.

- - - - - - - - - -

Exchanges for one serving of the entire menu equal ½ Milk, ½ B Vegetable, 2½ Fruit, 4 Bread, 5 Meat, 2 Fat.

* * * * *

Buffets for All Occasions

Menus and Recipes for Ten

Chicken Superb

Club Soda on Ice

Chicken Superb

Steamed Rice   **Green Peas**

Fruit Salad

D-Zerta Parfait

Chicken Superb (10 servings—2 pieces each)

5   large Chicken Breasts, halved
10   large Chicken Thighs
2   cans condensed Cream of Mushroom Soup
1½   cups dry Bread Crumbs
¼   cup Water
Salt and Pepper

Remove moisture from meat with paper towels. Mix water and cream of mushroom soup. Coat each piece of chicken with soup mixture, then dip in bread crumbs. Place in shallow baking dish; salt and pepper to taste. Add balance of soup mixture. Bake uncovered in 300-degree oven for 1 hour. Serve drippings over the chicken.

One serving equals 1 Bread Exchange, 3 Meat Exchanges, 1 Fat Exchange.

Steamed Rice (10 servings—1 cup each)

Cook 3 cups of rice according to directions on package. Serve hot, either on platter or in one-cup portions under the chicken.

One serving equals 2 Bread Exchanges.

Green Peas (10 servings—¹/₂ cup each)

4   *10-ounce packages frozen small Green Peas*
10   *teaspoons Margarine*

Cook peas according to directions on packages, then add margarine.

One serving equals 1 B Vegetable Exchange, 1 Fat Exchange.

Fruit Salad (10 servings—1 cup each)

2   *cups fresh Oranges, peeled and cut fine*
2   *cups unsweetened Pineapple Tidbits*
3   *medium Apples, chopped*
3   *small Bananas, sliced*

Chill pineapple and orange in a mixing bowl. Drain just before serving. Add bananas and apples, and mix gently. Serve cold on lettuce leaf.

One serving equals 2 Fruit Exchanges.

D-Zerta Parfait (10 servings — 1 parfait each)

   3   *packages Raspberry or Cherry D-Zerta*
   2   *cups Jane's Topping**

Prepare Jane's Topping.
Prepare D-Zerta according to directions on package. Dice the chilled and jelled D-Zerta. Build parfaits with alternating layers of D-Zerta and Jane's Topping. Keep in refrigerator until time to serve.
Parfait with topping equals Zero Exchange.

- - - - - - - - - -

Exchanges for one serving of the entire menu equal 1 B Vegetable, 2 Fruit, 3 Bread, 3 Meat, 2 Fat.

* * * * *

*Use recipe for Jane's Topping given in Part IV (see Index).

Pizza

Grape-Lemon Punch

Hot Popcorn   **Bacon-Onion Dip**

Pizza

Assorted Raw Vegetables

Vanilla Ice Cream - Coconut Topping

Grape-Lemon Punch (10 servings — 1 cup each)

    $2^1/_2$ cups unsweetened Grape Juice
    $1^1/_4$ cups Lemon Juice
    $2^1/_2$ teaspoons liquid Sucaryl
    7   cups Water (plain or carbonated)

Combine all ingredients; chill well; serve cold.
One serving equals 1 Fruit Exchange.

Hot Popcorn (10 servings — 1 cup each)

    $^1/_2$ cup raw Popcorn*

STOVE METHOD: Put popcorn in large saucepan. Place over medium-hot heat. To prevent corn from burning, shake saucepan constantly until all corn seems to be popped.

POPPER METHOD: Use only a popper that has a stirrer. Stir constantly, for popcorn cooked without oil burns easily.

Salt slightly. Serve hot.
One serving equals 1 Bread Exchange.

*This amount may make more than 10 cups of popped corn.

Bacon-Onion Dip (10 servings — scant ¹/₃ cup each)

2   packages dry Bacon-Onion Dip Mix
1¹/₂ cups Cottage Cheese
¹/₂   cup Buttermilk
¹/₂   cup imitation Sour Cream
3   ounces Cream Cheese
Salt

Blend buttermilk and cottage cheese in blender until smooth. Remove from blender and mix in other ingredients, adding salt to taste.

One serving equals 1 Meat Exchange.

Pizza (10 servings — 2 muffin halves each)

10   English Muffins, split in half
2   pounds lean ground Beef
10   ounces Mozzarelli Cheese
1   can (6-ounce) Tomato Paste
¹/₂   cup Hot Water
1¹/₂ teaspoons Salt
3   teaspoons Oregano

Using fresh muffins at room temperature, roll each half muffin with a rolling pin until it is flat and a little larger than its original size.

Sauté beef lightly. Add 1 teaspoon salt and 2 teaspoons oregano, and stir. Spread equal amounts of beef on all muffin halves. Cut cheese into thin slices and add ¹/₂ ounce to each muffin half on top of meat. Mix tomato paste, water, ¹/₂ teaspoon salt, and 1 teaspoon oregano; spread evenly on top of each piece. Bake in 425-degree oven for 8 to 10 minutes. Serve very hot.

One serving equals 2 Bread Exchanges, 3 Meat Exchanges.

Assorted Raw Vegetables (10 servings — any amount)

Use celery, carrot sticks, sliced zucchini, green pepper, radish roses, scallions, and cauliflower segments. Provide assorted sizes and colors. Prepare the day before and put in plastic bags in refrigerator to crisp and chill. Heap all vegetables in one large container for serving.

One serving equals 1 A Vegetable Exchange, 1 B Vegetable Exchange.

Vanilla Ice Cream - Coconut Topping
(10 servings — 1/2 cup each)

    5   cups *Vanilla Ice Cream*
    10   tablespoons shredded *Coconut (for topping)*

Use recipe for ice cream given in Part IV (see Index). Because the recipe makes 4 cups of ice cream, the quantities may be increased by one-fourth to provide a total of 10 servings.

Portion the ice cream into individual glass dishes, sprinkle 1 tablespoon of shredded coconut over the top, and put in freezer until ready to serve.

One serving equals 3/4 Milk Exchange, 1/2 Fat Exchange.

- - - - - - - - - -

Exchanges for one serving of the entire menu equal 3/4 Milk, 1 A Vegetable, 1 B Vegetable, 1 Fruit, 3 Bread, 4 Meat, 1/2 Fat.

* * * * *

Beef and Macaroni Casserole

Caribbean Cooler

Beef and Macaroni Casserole

Cole Slaw

Buttered French Bread

Pumpkin Chiffon Pie

Caribbean Cooler (10 servings — ³/₄ cup each)

1	medium-sized Banana, sliced
1	tablespoon Lemon Juice
3	cups unsweetened Pineapple Juice
1	teaspoon Vanilla Flavoring
1	teaspoon Coconut Flavoring
1¹/₂	teaspoons granulated Sucaryl
1¹/₂	cups Orange Juice
2	cups Club Soda

Mix all ingredients thoroughly in blender. Pour over ice in chilled glasses.

One serving equals 1¹/₂ Fruit Exchanges.

Beef and Macaroni Casserole (10 servings — 1 cup each)

2¹/₂ pounds lean ground Beef
3   cups Elbow Macaroni
¹/₂   cup minced Green Pepper
3¹/₂ cups Water
1   cup chopped Onions
3   teaspoons Salt
¹/₂   teaspoon Garlic Powder
4   cups canned Tomatoes

Lightly sauté beef, green pepper, and onion. Add uncooked macaroni, salt, and garlic powder; mix and continue cooking for 10 minutes, stirring constantly. Add tomatoes and water. Pour into large casserole and bake in 325-degree oven for 45 minutes.

One serving equals ¹/₂ B Vegetable Exchange, 1 Bread Exchange, 3 Meat Exchanges.

Cole Slaw (10 servings — about 1 cup each)

1   firm 3-pound Cabbage, chopped
1   cup Evaporated Milk
1   teaspoon Salt
2   teaspoons liquid Sucaryl
2   tablespoons Celery Seed
¹/₄   cup Vinegar

Mix together all ingredients except cabbage. When ready to serve pour mixture over cabbage and stir.

One serving equals ¹/₄ Milk Exchange, 1 A Vegetable Exchange.

Buttered French Bread (10 servings — 1 slice each)

10   medium slices French Bread
10   teaspoons Margarine

Spread 1 teaspoon margarine on each slice of bread and wrap all together in loaf shape in aluminum foil. Put in 325-degree oven for 20 minutes. Serve hot.

One serving equals 1 Bread Exchange, 1 Fat Exchange.

Pumpkin Chiffon Pie
(¹/₅ of 9-inch pie per serving; 2 pies needed)

2	baked 9-inch Pie Shells
3	cups canned Pumpkin
1	cup Milk
6	Eggs, separated
2	tablespoons Gelatin
¹/₂	cup cold Water
2	tablespoons liquid Sucaryl
1	teaspoon Ginger
1	teaspoon Nutmeg
1	teaspoon Cinnamon
1	teaspoon Salt

Sprinkle gelatin on cold water and let it stand 5 minutes. Put egg yolks in top of double boiler and beat slightly while they're cooking. Add pumpkin, milk, spices, salt, and Sucaryl. Cook until thick. Stir in soaked gelatin; cool thoroughly. Fold in egg whites that have been beaten stiff. Pour into pie shells and place in refrigerator.

One serving equals 1 Milk Exchange, 1 Bread Exchange, 3 Fat Exchanges.

- - - - - - - - - -

Exchanges for one serving of the entire menu equal 1¹/₄ Milk, 1 A Vegetable, ¹/₂ B Vegetable, 1¹/₂ Fruit, 3 Bread, 3 Meat, 4 Fat.

* * * * *

Meat Patties Wrapped in Bacon

Fresh Citrus Frappé

Meat Patties Wrapped in Bacon

Twice-Baked Potato   **Green Beans**

Tomato and Lettuce Salad

Pineapple Cheese Cake

Fresh Citrus Frappé (10 servings — ³/₄ cup each)

    2   Grapefruit, sectioned
    4   cups unsweetened Grapefruit Juice
    1¹/₂ teaspoons liquid Sucaryl

Remove white membrane from grapefruit. Put grapefruit sections in blender with juice and Sucaryl; blend until frothy. Pour into chilled glasses over ice.
One serving equals 1 Fruit Exchange.

Meat Patties Wrapped in Bacon
(10 servings — 3 ounces meat plus one strip bacon each)

    2¹/₂ pounds lean ground Beef
    10   strips Bacon
    Salt and Pepper

Salt and pepper meat. Form 10 equal patties of such a size that the bacon strips will just meet around them. Secure bacon with toothpicks. Broil and serve hot.
One serving equals 3 Meat Exchanges, 1 Fat Exchange.

Twice-Baked Potato (10 servings — 1/2 potato each)

> 5   large baking Potatoes
> 6   tablespoons Margarine
> 1   cup Hot Milk
> Salt and Pepper

Bake potatoes in 350-degree oven for 1¼ hours. Cut potatoes in half lengthwise while they're still hot. Scoop out potatoes, placing scoopings in large mixing bowl; add margarine and salt. Mash with mixer or hand masher and gradually add milk until smooth. Add more salt if desired. Repack whipped potatoes in shells; sprinkle tops with paprika if desired. The potatoes may be made in advance and stored in refrigerator or freezer. When ready to use, bring them to room temperature, then heat in 400-degree oven for 20 minutes or until slightly brown.

One serving equals 2 Bread Exchanges, 2 Fat Exchanges.

Green Beans (10 servings — 1/2 cup each)

> 3   cans Green Beans (1-pound size)
> 1/2 teaspoon Butter Flavoring

Boil beans in their own juice for 5 minutes. Drain, reserving 1 tablespoon of liquid. Add butter flavoring to the reserved liquid and mix with beans. Add a pinch of sweet basil or thyme if desired.

One serving equals 1 A Vegetable Exchange.

Tomato and Lettuce Salad (10 servings — 1 cup each)

> 1   firm head of Lettuce
> 5   medium-sized Tomatoes
> 2   tablespoons Mayonnaise
> Salt and Pepper

Break lettuce into bite-size pieces; add tomatoes chopped fine. Cover and refrigerate. Just before serving, add mayonnaise and stir well. Serve individually or in a large bowl.

One serving equals 1 A Vegetable Exchange, ½ Fat Exchange.

Pineapple Cheesecake
(10 servings—one-fifth of cheesecake each)

24	ounces creamed Cottage Cheese
2	3-ounce packages Cream Cheese
2	cups unsweetened Pineapple Tidbits, drained
2	tablespoons Gelatin
2	Eggs
8	teaspoons Lemon Juice
5	tablespoons liquid Sucaryl
2	teaspoons Vanilla Flavoring
10	drops Yellow Food-Coloring

Stir cottage cheese and cream cheese in blender. Dissolve gelatin in pineapple juice. Combine all ingredients and blend until smooth. Pour into 9-inch pie pans and bake in 350-degree oven for 30 minutes. Cool and refrigerate.

Topping for Cheesecake

3	cups unsweetened crushed Pineapple
8	teaspoons Cornstarch
8	teaspoons liquid Sucaryl
4	tablespoons Lemon Juice
8	drops Yellow Food-Coloring

Combine crushed pineapple, lemon juice, and cornstarch. Bring to a boil and cook 1 minute. Stir in food coloring and Sucaryl. Let cool thoroughly before spreading on top of cake.

One serving of cheesecake and topping equals ½ Milk Exchange, 1 Fruit Exchange, 1 Meat Exchange.

- - - - - - - - - -

Exchanges for one serving of the entire menu equal ½ Milk, 2 A Vegetable, 2 Fruit, 2 Bread, 4 Meat, 3½ Fat.

* * * * *

Baked Ham

Fruit Punch

Baked Ham

Pickled Beets   **Brussels Sprouts**

Pineapple-Pumpkin Fruit

Celery-Apple Salad

Buttered Rolls

Chocolate Pudding

Fruit Punch (10 servings—8 ounces each)

    1   quart Apple-Flavored Diet Drink
    1   quart Diet Ginger Ale
    2   cups Orange Juice
    ¼   cup Lemon Juice

   Place orange juice in freezer trays to make orange ice cubes. Combine lemon juice and apple drink with the frozen orange cubes and stir in blender until mushy. Stir in cold ginger ale. If desired add a little liquid Sucaryl for sweetness.
   One serving equals Zero Exchange.

Baked Ham (10 servings — 3 ounces each)

> 2   pounds cooked Ham
> Prepared Mustard

Slice ham into 3-ounce servings. Lay slices together on shallow pan, so that they can be heated without drying. Spread mustard over top of ham, if desired. Place in 350-degree oven for 15 minutes. Arrange on serving platter; garnish with parsley.
One serving equals 3 Meat Exchanges.

Pickled Beets (10 servings — 1/2 cup each)

> 5   cups julienne-cut canned Beets
> 1   cup Cider Vinegar
> 2   tablespoons grated Onion
> 1   clove Garlic, mashed
> 2   teaspoons liquid Sucaryl

Mix all seasonings. Drain beets and add to seasonings. Allow to marinate 24 hours. When ready to serve remove garlic bits.
One serving equals 1 B Vegetable Exchange.

Brussels Sprouts (10 servings — 4 sprouts each)

> Frozen Brussels Sprouts (enough packages to provide a
>   total of 40 sprouts)
> 1/4   teaspoon Butter Flavoring

Cook sprouts according to directions on package(s). Drain. Season with butter flavoring mixed with small amount of cooking liquid. Serve hot. (Do not allow to stand before serving because flavor and appearance will deteriorate.)
One serving equals 1 A Vegetable Exchange.

Pineapple—Pumpkin Fruit (10 servings — ³/₄ cup each)

1	can Solid-Pack Pumpkin (about 29 ounces)
1	cup unsweetened Crushed Pineapple
1	cup Buttermilk
1	Egg, separated
1	teaspoon Lemon Juice
1	teaspoon Cinnamon
¹/₄	teaspoon Nutmeg
³/₈	teaspoon liquid Sucaryl
2	teaspoons Vanilla Flavoring
¹/₂	teaspoon Salt

Place 1 cup pumpkin, all of pineapple, ¹/₂ cup buttermilk, cinnamon, nutmeg, Sucaryl, egg yolk, and vanilla flavoring in blender and blend until smooth. Slowly add remaining pumpkin and remaining buttermilk. Continue blending until smooth. Fold in beaten egg white. Pour mixture into baking dish and bake, uncovered, for 45 minutes in 325-degree oven. Serve warm.

One serving equals 1 B Vegetable Exchange.

Celery-Apple Salad (10 servings — ³/₄ cup each)

4	medium-sized unpeeled Apples, chopped
3	ribs Celery, chopped fine
¹/₂	cup Evaporated Milk
¹/₄	cup Cider Vinegar
³/₄	teaspoon liquid Sucaryl
¹/₈	teaspoon Salt
1	teaspoon Celery Seed

Combine milk, Sucaryl, salt, vinegar, and celery seed; mix thoroughly. A bit more salt, sweetener, or vinegar may be added if desired. Serve on lettuce leaf.

One serving equals 1 Fruit Exchange.

Buttered Rolls (10 servings — 1 roll each)

    10   small Rolls
    10   teaspoons Margarine

Split each roll and spread with 1 teaspoon margarine. Heat and serve hot.

One serving equals 1 Bread Exchange, 1 Fat Exchange.

Chocolate Pudding (10 servings — 1/2 cup each)

    2¹/₂   tablespoons Gelatin
    5   cups Milk
    6   tablespoons Cocoa
    3   tablespoons liquid Sucaryl
    1¹/₂   teaspoons Vanilla Flavoring
    ¹/₄   teaspoon Salt

Soften gelatin in 1 cup milk and set aside for a few minutes. Mix the cocoa with 1/4 cup milk, then gradually add the rest of the milk and heat until simmering. Add gelatin mixture and stir well. Combine with remaining ingredients and pour into individual dessert dishes.

One serving equals 1/2 Milk Exchange.

- - - - - - - - - -

Exchanges for one serving of the entire menu equal 1/2 Milk, 1 A Vegetable, 2 B Vegetable, 1 Fruit, 1 Bread, 3 Meat, 1 Fat.

* * * * *

SEATED DINNERS

Teenagers or young adults? Whichever label is attached the group remains the same the world over—charming, teasing, perturbed at times, yet always fun. Its members are notorious for "horsing around." They resist most attempts at formality, but as they grow older they will agree to go along with your ideas for a seated dinner party in celebration of a special occasion, such as the end of the football season, a graduation, a birthday, or a holiday.

If the dinner is for teammates and their dates, school colors can be used in the decorations along with sports equipment, such as tennis rackets and nets, a baseball bat, or a basketball. For winter parties, sprigs of mistletoe can be placed over the doorways.

The young person hosting the party should be allowed to choose the entertainment. If dancing is decided upon, he or she should select the records to be played. Charades might be chosen as a good icebreaker. If attendance at a movie, either before or after the dinner, is elected, and if the guests are old enough, they should be allowed to go alone while the parents remain at home, letting their son or daughter play host.

Menus and Recipes for Four

Chicken-Rice Casserole

Chicken-Rice Casserole

Broccoli **Cranberry Relish**

Baby Carrots

Fruit Delight

Chicken-Rice Casserole (4 servings—1 cup each)

1   cup cooked Chicken or Turkey cut in bite-size pieces
1/2   small can chopped Mushrooms
1/2   cup toasted Bread Crumbs
3/4   cup cooked Rice
1/2   teaspoon grated Onion
2   tablespoons Margarine
3   tablespoons Flour
1   cup Milk
1/2   cup Chicken Broth
4   ounces Cheddar Cheese, grated
Salt
Celery Salt
Paprika

Melt margarine, add flour, and stir until smooth. Add milk and broth (fat removed). Blend in cheese. Add remaining ingredients except bread crumbs. Place half of crumbs in bottom of casserole or baking dish, then pour in chicken mixture. Sprinkle remaining crumbs on top, then sprinkle with paprika and celery salt. Bake in 350-degree oven for 30 minutes, or until bubbly.

One serving equals 1 Bread Exchange, 3 Meat Exchanges, 1½ Fat Exchanges.

Broccoli (4 servings — 3 spears each)

½	bunch fresh Broccoli
¼	teaspoon Lemon Juice
½	teaspoon Butter Flavoring

Trim broccoli carefully, allowing three medium-sized spears per person. Steam in small amount of salted water about 10 minutes, until just tender. Drain, reserving 2 tablespoons of liquid. Keep broccoli hot. Mix the reserved liquid, the butter flavoring, and the lemon juice; pour over hot broccoli.

One serving equals 1 A Vegetable Exchange.

Cranberry Relish (4 servings — ¼ cup each)

½	cup Orange pieces
1	cup raw Cranberries
¾	tablespoon liquid Sucaryl

Cut orange into small pieces, removing the seeds but not the peeling. Whip the orange pieces in a blender until the large pieces are broken up. Add Sucaryl and cranberries and continue blending for a short time.

One serving equals Zero Exchange.

Baby Carrots (4 servings — ½ cup each)

2	cups thinly sliced baby Carrots
½	cup Chicken Bouillon
¼	teaspoon Accent
1	teaspoon Salt
2	tablespoons chopped Parsley
¼	teaspoon Butter Flavoring
¼	teaspoon Oregano
	Pepper

Place all ingredients except parsley and oregano into a large pan with tight lid and bring to a boil. Simmer for 15 minutes, or until carrots are tender. Pour off most of excess liquid, add parsley and oregano. Serve immediately.

One serving equals 1 B Vegetable Exchange.

Fruit Delight (4 servings — 1 cup each)

    1   cup red D-Zerta gelatin, prepared and cut into small cubes
    ½   tablespoon unflavored Gelatin
    ¼   cup Orange Juice
    1   cup unsweetened Pineapple, cubed
    ½   cup finely grated Coconut
    1   cup Jane's Topping*

Soak unflavored gelatin in orange juice for 5 minutes. Heat very gently until dissolved, then cool to room temperature. Add pineapple, coconut, D-Zerta cubes, and topping. Mix gently.

One serving (fruit delight with topping) equals 1 Fruit Exchange, 1 Fat Exchange.

- - - - - - - - - -

Exchanges for one serving of the entire menu equal 1 A Vegetable, 1 B Vegetable, 1 Fruit, 1 Bread, 3 Meat, 2½ Fat.

* * * * *

*Use the recipe for Jane's Topping given in Part IV (see Index), but cut the amounts in half.

Veal Cutlets

Veal Cutlets
Potatoes in Cream Sauce   **Spinach**
Baked Apple   **Banana Cookies**

Veal Cutlets (4 servings—3 ounces each)

4   4-ounce Veal Cutlets
4   teaspoons Cooking Oil
1   Egg
1   cup dry Bread Crumbs
Salt and Pepper

Beat egg with 1 tablespoon of water. Dip each cutlet in egg mixture, then in bread crumbs. Sprinkle with salt and pepper. Heat the cooking oil in an iron or no-stick skillet; place the breaded cutlets in the skillet over medium heat. Continue cooking until the cutlets are "fork" tender. Serve hot.

One serving equals 1 Bread Exchange, 3 Meat Exchanges, 1 Fat Exchange.

Potatoes in Cream Sauce (4 servings—1 cup each)

2   medium-sized Potatoes
2   cups Skim Milk
1/2   teaspoon Salt
1   dash Pepper
3   teaspoons Flour
4   teaspoons Margarine
1   dash Paprika

Peel potatoes and cube them. Cook until tender (about 20 minutes) in salted water. Drain. Blend margarine and flour over medium heat. Add milk and cook until thickened. Add salt and cubed potatoes. Season to taste with salt and pepper. Add a dash of paprika, and serve hot.

One serving equals ½ Milk Exchange, 1½ Bread Exchanges, 1 Fat Exchange.

Spinach (4 servings — ¾ cup each)

1	package (10 ounces) fresh Spinach
½	teaspoon Butter Flavoring
½	teaspoon Lemon Juice

Salt and Pepper

Cook spinach in half a cup of water until tender (about 15 minutes). When ready to serve, add butter flavoring and lemon juice, then sprinkle lightly with salt and pepper.

One serving equals 1 A Vegetable Exchange.

Baked Apple (4 servings — 1 apple each)

4	medium-sized cooking Apples
¾	cup Water
2	tablespoons granulated Sucaryl
¼	teaspoon Nutmeg
¼	teaspoon Cinnamon

Peel a wide circle around the middle of each apple, and remove core. Place each apple in an individual baking dish. Mix other ingredients and pour mixture over apples. Bake, uncovered, in 325-degree oven for 45 minutes. Remove from oven and serve at room temperature.

One serving equals 1½ Fruit Exchanges.

Banana Cookies (4 servings—2 cookies each)*

2	ounces Margarine
1½	cups All-Purpose Flour
⅔	cup granulated Sucaryl
1	Banana
1	Egg
2	teaspoons Vanilla Flavoring
1	teaspoon Baking Powder
⅛	teaspoon Salt

Sift flour, Sucaryl, baking powder, and salt into a mixing bowl; add softened margarine and mix well. Mash the banana with a fork and combine with vanilla flavoring and egg. Add to first mixture and mix well. Drop by teaspoonfuls on ungreased cookie sheet. Bake in 350-degree oven for about 20 minutes. When done remove from cookie sheet with a spatula.

One serving (2 cookies) equals ½ Bread Exchange, 1 Fat Exchange.

- - - - - - - - - -

Exchanges for one serving of the entire menu equal ½ Milk, 1 A Vegetable, 1½ Fruit, 3 Bread, 3 Meat, 3 Fat.

* * * * *

*This recipe makes about 3 dozen cookies; there will be many left over for future use.

Spagetti with Meat Sauce

Spaghetti with Meat Sauce

Tossed Green Salad

Frozen Lemon Pie

Spaghetti with Meat Sauce
(4 servings — 1 cup spaghetti plus 1 cup sauce for each)

1   *pound lean ground Beef*
1/2   *pound Spaghetti*
4   *ounces Tomato Paste*
1 1/2 *teaspoons Salt*
1   *clove Garlic, crushed*
1/2   *teaspoon Oregano*
1/4   *teaspoon Sweet Basil*
1/4   *teaspoon liquid Sucaryl*
1/2   *teaspoon Onion Powder*
1   *Bay Leaf*
1/4   *teaspoon Rosemary*
2   *cups Water*
Shaker of Parmesan Cheese

Brown meat over medium heat in a large heavy pot. Add tomato paste. Stir and let fry with meat for a few seconds. Add all ingredients except spaghetti and parmesan cheese. Mix well. Simmer for 2 hours. Add water if too thick; volume should be about 4 cups.

Cook spaghetti according to directions on package. Drain. Serve one cup of the plain spaghetti on a plate; pour or ladle one cup of the sauce over this. Provide container of grated Parmesan cheese for sprinkling on top.

One serving equals 1 B Vegetable Exchange, 2 Bread Exchanges, 3 Meat Exchanges.

Tossed Green Salad (4 servings—1 cup each)

$1/2$ head Romaine
$1/2$ head Bibb Lettuce
4   leaves Spinach

After washing greens, pat dry with paper towels, tear into bite-size pieces, and store in refrigerator in plastic container until ready to mix salad. Provide oil-and-vinegar dressing (recipe follows).

Oil-and-Vinegar Dressing (4 servings—1 tablespoon each)

8   teaspoons Salad Oil
4   teaspoons Vinegar
$1/4$ teaspoon Salad Herbs
Salt and Pepper
Garlic Salt (optional)

Mix all ingredients thoroughly.   Pour dressing over cold greens just before serving.

One serving (greens with dressing) equals 1 A Vegetable Exchange, 2 Fat Exchanges.

Frozen Lemon Pie (4 servings—each 2 by $3^{1}/_{4}$ inches)*

2   Eggs, separated
1   Lemon (juice and grated rind)
$1/8$ teaspoon Salt
2   teaspoons liquid Sucaryl
$1^{1}/_{2}$ cups Cool Whip
12   Graham Crackers, crushed

*The Recipe makes 6 servings; there will be 2 left over.)

Beat egg yolks well. Add lemon juice, grated rind, salt, and Sucaryl. Cook in top of double boiler until mixture coats spoon, stirring constantly. Cool. Fold in Cool Whip and stiffly beaten egg whites. Sprinkle half of crumbs over the bottom of a refrigerator ice tray that has been lined with wax paper. Pour custard over crumbs and cover with remaining crumbs. Freeze until firm; cut into 6 servings.

One serving equals ½ Milk Exchange, 1 Bread Exchange.

- - - - - - - - - -

Exchanges for one serving of the entire menu equal ½ Milk, 1 A Vegetable, 1 B Vegetable, 3 Bread, 3 Meat, 2 Fat.

* * * * *

Oven-Fried Fish

Oven-Fried Fish

Tomatoes and Macaroni

Green Peas and Celery

Lettuce Wedge - Thousand Island Dressing

Cherry Upside-Down Cake

Oven-Fried Fish (4 servings—3 ounces each)

1   *pound White Fish Fillets*
¼   *cup Flour*
½   *teaspoon Paprika*
4   *teaspoons Cooking Oil*
Salt and Pepper
1 Lemon

Divide fillets into 4-ounce portions and pat dry with paper towels. Spray a shallow baking dish with PAM. Mix flour and paprika. Roll each fillet in flour mix, then place on baking dish. Brush with oil; sprinkle with salt and pepper. Bake uncovered in a 300-degree oven for 15 to 20 minutes. Serve hot with a wedge of lemon on the side.

One serving equals 3 Meat Exchanges, 1 Fat Exchange.

Tomatoes and Macaroni (4 servings — 1 cup each)

4   cups cooked Macaroni
2   tablespoons Margarine
1   can Tomatoes (14 ounces)
1   small Onion, diced
Salt and Pepper

Sauté onion in margarine until clear. Mash the tomatoes; add seasonings, macaroni, and onion. Simmer about 20 minutes until flavors are well blended.

One serving equals 1 A Vegetable Exchange, 2 Bread Exchanges, 1½ Fat Exchanges.

Green Peas and Celery (4 servings — ³/₄ cup each)

2   cups canned small Green Peas
1   cup cooked Celery, diced
¹/₈   teaspoon Soy Sauce
¹/₄ .   teaspoon Butter Flavoring
Salt and Pepper

Drain liquids from heated peas and from cooked celery. Combine all ingredients. Let flavors blend for a few minutes. Serve hot.

One serving equals 1 B Vegetable Exchange.

Lettuce Wedge with Thousand Island Dressing
(4 servings — ¹/₄ head lettuce with dressing for each)

1   small head Lettuce

Core, wash, and trim lettuce. Store in refrigerator until ready to serve, then cut in quarters.

Thousand Island Dressing
(4 servings — 1 heaping tablespoon each)

2	tablespoons Mayonnaise
1½	hard boiled Eggs
2	tablespoons sugar-free Dill Pickles, chopped fine
1	teaspoon Tomato Paste
1	teaspoon Vinegar
⅛	teaspoon liquid Sucaryl

Combine all ingredients except eggs. Mix well and let stand a few minutes. Chop eggs fine and add to mixture. Add a little more seasoning if desired. Serve 1 heaping tablespoon over each quarter-head of lettuce.

One serving (lettuce and dressing) equals 1 A Vegetable Exchange, 2 Fat Exchanges.

Cherry Upside Down Cake (4 servings — ¼ recipe each)

2	cups tart Red Cherries
1	cup plus 2 tablespoons granulated Sucaryl
1	tablespoon Margarine
1	Egg
½	cup plus 2 tablespoons Flour
⅛	teaspoon Salt
¼	cup Milk
⅛	teaspoon Almond Flavoring
1	teaspoon Baking Powder

Drain cherries and save juice for making cherry sauce. Spread cherries over bottom of greased shallow loaf pan. Sprinkle 1 cup granulated Sucaryl over cherries. Cream margarine with 2 tablespoons granulated Sucaryl; add egg and beat well. Mix and sift flour, baking powder, and salt. Add alternately with milk to first mixture, then add flavoring. Pour batter over cherries and bake in 350-degree oven for 20 to 25 minutes. Serve warm with cherry sauce (recipe follows).

Cherry Sauce (4 servings — ¹/₄ recipe each)

    Cherry Juice from Cake Cherries
¹/₂   *tablespoon Corn Starch*
1   *tablespoon Water*
¹/₄   *cup granulated Sucaryl*
2   *drops Almond Flavoring*

Mix cornstarch, water, cherry juice, and Sucaryl. Heat and boil 2 minutes. Add almond flavoring. Serve warm over cherry cake.

One serving (cake and sauce) equals 1 Fruit Exchange, 1 Bread Exchange, 1 Fat Exchange. (Sauce contains Zero Exchange.)

- - - - - - - - - -

Exchanges for one serving of the entire menu equal 2 A Vegetable, 1 B Vegetable, 1 Fruit, 3 Bread, 3 Meat, 5¹/₂ Fat.

* * * * *

Skillet Beef and Noodles

Skillet Beef and Noodles

Whole Kernel Corn　　　**Buttered Green Beans**

Celery and Carrot Sticks

Banana Refresher

Skillet Beef and Noodles (4 servings — 2 cups each)

1　　pound lean ground Beef
2　　cups raw Noodles
1/4　teaspoon Pepper
1　　envelope dry Onion Soup Mix
1　　can Tomatoes (14 ounces)
Salt

Cook noodles according to directions on package. Brown beef in skillet. Stir in remaining ingredients and cover. Cook for 20 minutes on low heat. Add more seasoning if desired. Serve hot.

One serving equals 1 A Vegetable Exchange, 2 Bread Exchanges, 3 Meat Exchanges.

Whole Kernel Corn (4 servings — 2/3 cup each)

2 2/3　cups canned Whole Kernel Corn
4　　teaspoons Margarine
Salt and Pepper

Heat corn in its own juice until simmering; drain and measure corn kernels. Add margarine, salt, and pepper. Serve hot.
One serving equals 2 Bread Exchanges, 1 Fat Exchange.

Buttered Green Beans (4 servings — 1/2 cup each)

2   cups cooked Green Beans
4   teaspoons Margarine
Salt
1   pinch of Sweet Basil

Add seasonings to beans, heat slowly while stirring until all ingredients are blended. Serve hot.
One serving equals 1 A Vegetable Exchange, 1 Fat Exchange.

Celery and Carrot Sticks (4 servings)

2   ribs Celery
2   medium-sized Carrots

Trim and scrape carrots; cut into strips. Scrub celery, divide into strips. Store in refrigerator in plastic bag until ready to use.
One serving equals 1 A Vegetable Exchange.

Banana Refresher (4 servings — 1 1/4 cups each)

3   small Bananas, sliced
2   teaspoons Lemon Juice
1 1/2   cups Buttermilk
1 1/2   cups Milk
1   teaspoon liquid Sucaryl
1/2   teaspoon Vanilla Flavoring
1/2   cup crushed Ice

Put sliced bananas in blender, add lemon juice, and blend. Add remaining ingredients and blend at high speed until frothy. Serve in parfait glasses, with spoon or large straw.

One serving equals ½ Milk Exchange, 2 Fruit Exchanges.

- - - - - - - - - -

Exchanges for one serving of the entire menu equal ½ Milk, 3 A Vegetable, 2 Fruit, 4 Bread, 3 Meat, 2 Fat.

* * * * *

PART III

Parties for the Diabetic

Adult

COOKOUTS

For pioneers pressing westward in covered wagons, cooking out-of-doors was a necessity. For present-day households it has become a social ritual enjoyed by young and old. The charm of campfires and the tantalizing aroma of food grilled over coals always stimulate the imagination as well as the appetite.

Cookouts can be informal and casual or formal and sophisticated, or variations of either type. Cooking is done on a grill of appropriate type for the setting—one's backyard, a balcony of an apartment complex, a park, a campsite. Wherever the cookout is held, remember to

KEEP HOT FOODS HOT

AND

COLD FOODS COLD

Menus and Recipes for Eight

Weiners on Buns

Lemon-Lime Drink

Weiners on Buns

Baked Beans

Cole Slaw

Chocolate Sundae

Lemon-Lime Drink (8 servings — 1 cup each)

2   quarts diet Lemon-Lime Soda

Chill soda until very cold. Serve in tall glasses with ice cubes. Garnish with fresh mint, if available.
One serving equals Zero Exchange.

Weiners on Buns (8 servings — 2 each)

16   small Weiners
16   Hot-Dog Buns
Prepared Mustard

Roast weiners over hot coals; serve each on warmed bun, with mustard if desired.
One serving equals 2 Meat Exchanges, 2 Bread Exchanges.

Baked Beans (8 servings — 1/2 cup each)

4   cups cooked Navy Beans
1/2   cup unsweetened Ketchup
3   tablespoons grated Onion
1   teaspoon Liquid Smoke
1   teaspoon Worcestershire Sauce
1/2   teaspoon Accent
1   teaspoon Salt
1/4   teaspoon Pepper

Combine all ingredients and place in casserole. Bake in 350-degree oven for 30 minutes.
One serving equals 2 Bread Exchanges.

Cole Slaw (8 servings — 1 cup each)

1   firm 3-pound Cabbage
1 1/2 cups canned Skim Milk
5   tablespoons Mayonnaise
3 1/2 tablespoons Vinegar
2   teaspoons liquid Sucaryl
2   tablespoons Celery Seed
1   teaspoon Salt

Combine all ingredients except cabbage, and mix well. Shred cabbage, or chop fine. Just before serving pour the liquid dressing over the cabbage and stir.
One serving equals 1/2 Milk Exchange, 1 A Vegetable Exchange, 1 Fat Exchange.

Chocolate Sundae (8 servings — 1/2 cup ice cream each)

Use recipe for ice cream given in Part IV (see Index).

Chocolate Syrup for Sundae
(8 servings — 2¹/₂ tablespoons each)

    1¹/₂ cups Evaporated Milk
    ¹/₂   cup unsweetened Cocoa
    3   teaspoons liquid Sucaryl
    1   teaspoon Vanilla Flavoring
    ¹/₈   teaspoon Salt

Combine the cocoa with 4 tablespoons milk; mix until smooth. If necessary, add more milk to make a paste. Add the rest of the milk very slowly. Add salt and cook until mixture comes to a boil. Immediately turn heat to simmer and cook mixture until it thickens. Cool and add the Sucaryl; mix thoroughly.

One serving of ice cream alone (¹/₂ cup) equals ³/₄ Milk Exchange. One serving of chocolate syrup alone (2¹/₂ tablespoons) equals ¹/₂ Milk Exchange.

- - - - - - - - - -

Exchanges for one serving of the entire menu equal 1³/₄ Milk, 1 A Vegetable, 4 Bread, 2 Meat, 1 Fat.

* * * * *

Hamburger on Bun

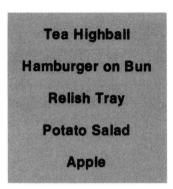

Tea Highball

Hamburger on Bun

Relish Tray

Potato Salad

Apple

Tea Highball (8 servings—1 cup each)

   4   cups double-strength Tea
   2   teaspoons Vanilla Flavoring
   1/2 teaspoon liquid Sucaryl (more or less, as desired)
   1/2 teaspoon Angostura Bitters
   Club Soda

Mix all ingredients except Club Soda. Put ice cubes in tall glasses, and divide the tea mixture among them. Fill glasses with soda water.

One serving equals Zero Exchange.

Hamburgers (8 servings—1 hamburger each)

   2   pounds lean ground Beef
   8   small Hamburger Buns
   Salt and Pepper

Mix meat, salt, and pepper; shape into eight patties of equal size. Cook on grill over hot coals, or broil in stove broiler.

One serving equals 1¹/₂ Bread Exchanges, 3 Meat Exchanges.

Relish Tray (8 servings)

> *Dill Pickle Slices*
> *Thin slices of Onions*
> *Radishes*
> *Sliced Tomatoes*
> *Lettuce Leaves*
> *Mustard*

One serving equals 1 A Vegetable Exchange.

Potato Salad (8 servings — ⁵/₈ cup each)

4	cups boiled Potatoes, diced
¹/₄	cup Vinegar
1	teaspoon Celery Seed
1	tablespoon Prepared Mustard
4	hard-boiled Eggs, chopped
1	Green Pepper, diced fine
1	stalk Celery
¹/₂	cup chopped Onion
5	tablespoons Mayonnaise
	Salt and Pepper
	Parsley, for garnish
3	Dill Pickles, chopped

Mix potatoes with vinegar and celery seed, and add chopped eggs. Allow to cool, then add remaining ingredients. Garnish with parsley and serve cold.

One serving equals ¹/₂ Bread Exchange, ¹/₂ Meat Exchange, 2 Fat Exchanges.

Apple (8 servings — 1 apple each)

   8   *Apples*

One serving (1 small apple, about 2 inches in diameter) equals 1 Fruit Exchange.

- - - - - - - - - -

Exchanges for one serving of the entire menu equal 1 A Vegetable, 1 Fruit, 2 Bread, 3½ Meat, 2 Fat.

* * * * *

Lamb Shish Kabobs

Chilled Consommé

Lamb Shish Kabobs

French Bread

Tossed Salad

Blue Cheese and Saltines

Chilled Consommé (8 servings — ½ cup each)

    3   cans Jellied Beef Consommé
    8   tablespoons Sour Cream
    8   wedges fresh Lemon
    8   teaspoons Caviar

Chill consommé over night. Divide it equally among eight old-fashion glasses, taking care to break it up as little as possible. Put 1 tablespoon sour cream, then 1 teaspoon caviar on top of each. Capers may be substituted if caviar is not available. Serve cold with lemon wedges.

One serving equals ½ Fat Exchange.

Lamb Shish Kabobs (8 servings—1 skewer each)

2	pounds meat from Leg of Lamb
2	cups Mushrooms
2	large Green Peppers
4	cups Cherry Tomatoes
1	Eggplant, peeled and cut into 1-inch cubes
2	cups small whole Onions
1	teaspoon Garlic Powder
1	teaspoon Mushroom Powder
3	tablespoons Salad Oil
1	cup Red Wine
$1/2$	teaspoon Oregano
$1/8$	teaspoon Rosemary
	Salt and Pepper

Cut meat into $1^1/_2$-inch cubes. Mix the dry seasonings with wine, vinegar, and salad oil. Marinate meat in this mixture over night and until ready to use. Thread the meat and vegetables alternately on long skewers. Cook over hot coals for a minute or two on each of the four sides. When cooking is done, place skewers on platter to serve. When serving, use the French bread described in the following recipe to push ingredients from skewers onto individual plates—one slice per skewer, leaving the slice on the plate.

One serving equals 1 A Vegetable Exchange, 1 B Vegetable Exchange, 3 Meat Exchanges, 1 Fat Exchange.

French Bread (8 servings—2 slices each)

16 slices French Bread, about $1^1/_2$ inches thick

Wrap sliced bread in aluminum foil and heat in oven. (Use eight of the slices for removing meat and vegetables from skewers, leaving the remaining slices wrapped in foil for later serving.)

One serving equals 2 Bread Exchanges.

Tossed Salad (8 servings—1 cup each)

1	small head Lettuce
1	bunch Spinach
1	Cucumber
4	Green Onions
6	Radishes
4	teaspoons Wine Vinegar
8	teaspoons Salad Oil
	Salt and Pepper

Wash lettuce and spinach carefully; shake, and dry with paper towels. Place in refrigerator hydrator to chill and crisp. Tear greens into bite-size pieces; slice cucumber, onions, and radishes. Toss all ingredients with oil and vinegar.

One serving equals 1 A Vegetable Exchange, 1 Fat Exchange.

Blue Cheese and Saltines
(8 servings—1 ounce cheese and 3 saltines each)

8	ounces Blue Cheese
24	Saltines

Divide cheese into 1-ounce servings. Serve on salad or bread-and-butter plate.

One serving equals ⅔ Bread Exchange, 1 Meat Exchange.

- - - - - - - - - -

Exchanges for one serving of the entire menu equal 2 A Vegetable, 1 B Vegetable, 2⅔ Bread, 4 Meat, 2½ Fat.

* * * * *

Barbecued Ribs

Orange Frappé

Barbecued Ribs

Baked Potato

Broccoli Salad

Prune Pudding with Lemon Sauce

Orange Frappé (8 servings — ³/₄ cup each)

2	cups Orange Sections
2	cups Orange Juice
¹/₈	teaspoon Angostura Bitters
8	Ice Cubes

Remove white membrane and seeds from orange sections. Put all ingredients into blender and blend at top speed only until ice is broken up. Serve immediately in well-chilled sherbet glasses.
One serving equals 1 Fruit Exchange.

Barbecued Ribs (8 servings — divided equally)

8   pounds lean Pork Ribs (no fat)
Salt and Pepper
Barbecue Sauce (recipe follows)

Parboil or steam ribs on stove top for 30 minutes. Sprinkle with salt and pepper. Place ribs on grill, not too close to coals. Watch carefully, turn frequently, brushing with barbecue sauce at each turning. Cook for about 30 minutes, or until ribs are well browned. Serve hot.

Barbecue Sauce for Ribs

   1/2   cup Tomato Paste
   1   cup Vinegar
   2   cups Hot Water
   2   tablespoons liquid Sucaryl
   1   tablespoon Garlic Salt
   1/2   teaspoon Black Pepper
   1   teaspoon Liquid Smoke
   1   tablespoon Meat Tenderizer

Mix all ingredients; simmer about 5 minutes.
One serving (ribs with sauce) equals 2 Meat Exchanges.

Baked Potatoes (8 servings — 1 potato each)

   8   medium-sized Potatoes
   16   teaspoons Margarine
   Salt and Pepper

Scrub potatoes and bake in 400-degree preheated oven for 1 1/4 hours. Wrap potato in kitchen towel and gently mash or knead to soften the potato before splitting lengthwise. Add salt, pepper, and 1 teaspoon margarine to each potato half. Serve hot.
One serving equals 2 Bread Exchanges, 2 Fat Exchanges.

Broccoli Salad (8 servings — 1 cup each)

   1   large bunch Broccoli
   4   medium-sized Tomatoes
   1   bunch Green Onions
   1/3   cup Mayonnaise
   2   tablespoons Lemon Juice
   Salt and Pepper

Use only fresh broccoli, not frozen. Cut broccoli into natural separations, lengthwise. With a sharp knife, peel lower part of each stem and cut in half lengthwise. Blanch in boiling water for 2 minutes. Drain well. Chill.

Cut broccoli into bite-size pieces; cut tomatoes into small wedges; slice green onions. Sliced radishes may be added, if desired. Combine mayonnaise, lemon juice, salt, and pepper; add to vegetables. Toss gently. Serve cold.

One serving equals 2 A Vegetable Exchanges, 2 Fat Exchanges.

Prune Pudding with Lemon Sauce (8 servings — $^2/_3$ cup each)

24	medium-sized dried Prunes
3	cups Milk
4	tablespoons Margarine
3	slices Bread, crumbled
$1^1/_2$	teaspoons liquid Sucaryl
$^3/_4$	teaspoon Cinnamon
$^1/_3$	teaspoon Nutmeg
$1^1/_2$	teaspoons Salt
$1^1/_2$	teaspoons Vanilla Flavoring
3	Eggs, slightly beaten
$1^1/_2$	teaspoons Lemon Juice
$^3/_4$	cup Lemon Sauce (recipe follows)

Place prunes in saucepan and cover with boiling water; with pan covered, simmer about 20 minutes, or until tender. Drain, saving juice. Remove pits. Chop pulp finely; add $^1/_4$ cup prune juice to chopped fruit. Scald milk, add remaining ingredients, and mix with chopped prunes. Turn into 9-inch casserole which has been sprayed with PAM. Set in pan of hot water in oven and bake at 350 degrees for 45 minutes.

Lemon Sauce for Pudding (8 servings — 1¹/₂ tablespoons each)

    3   *tablespoons Lemon Juice*
    1¹/₂ *tablespoons Cornstarch*
    1¹/₂ *tablespoons cold Water*
    1¹/₂ *cups boiling Water*
    3   *teaspoons Margarine*
    3   *teaspoons liquid Sucaryl*
    1   *small pinch of Salt*

Mix cornstarch and cold water thoroughly; add boiling water and boil for 5 minutes, stirring constantly. Remove from fire, cool slightly, and stir in remaining ingredients.

One serving (pudding with sauce) equals 1 Milk Exchange, 1¹/₂ Fruit Exchanges, 1 Fat Exchange.

- - - - - - - - - -

Exchanges for one serving of the entire menu equal 1 Milk, 2 A Vegetable, 2¹/₂ Fruit, 2 Bread, 2 Meat, 5 Fat.

* * * * *

Broiled Fish Fillets

Bouillon

Broiled Fish Fillets

Corn on Cob

Dill Pickle   **Celery**   **Sliced Tomato**

Deep-Dish Apple Pie

Bouillon (8 servings — 1 cup each)

    8   *Bouillon Cubes (fat free)*

Place one bouillon cube in each cup, add boiling water, and stir well. Serve hot.

One serving equals Zero Exchange.

Fish Fillet (8 servings — 3 ounces each)

    2   *pounds Fish Fillets*
    8   *teaspoons Cooking Oil*
    2   *Lemons*
    Salt and Pepper

Divide fish into eight equal portions. Rub with oil, salt, and pepper. Spray hinged wire grid with PAM; place fillets in grid and cook over coals until fish flakes, approximately 10 minutes, turning occasionally. Serve with wedges of lemon.

One serving equals 3 Meat Exchanges, 1 Fat Exchange.

Corn on Cob (8 servings — 1 ear each)

8   ears Corn, about 4 inches long (fresh or frozen)
8   teaspoons Margarine, in individual servings
Salt and Pepper

If corn is frozen, follow directions on package. If fresh corn is used, put 1 cup water in large pot and bring to a boil. Add corn and cook covered, for 10 minutes. Serve with salt and pepper and 1 teaspoon margarine.

One serving equals 1 Bread Exchange, 1 Fat Exchange.

Dill Pickle, Celery, Sliced Tomato (8 servings)

4   medium-sized Tomatoes
4   ribs Celery
4   medium-sized Dill Pickles

Quarter the tomatoes, cut celery into sticks, and slice pickles. Arrange on a platter.

One serving equals 1 A Vegetable Exchange.

Deep-Dish Apple Pie (8 servings — $^1/_8$ pie each)

4   cooking Apples, peeled and sliced
2   tablespoons Cornstarch
$^1/_2$ teaspoon Cinnamon
$^1/_4$ teaspoon Clove
$^1/_4$ cup Water
2   tablespoons Lemon Juice
2   teaspoons liquid Sucaryl
3   tablespoons Margarine

Mix cinnamon, clove, and cornstarch well. Toss with apple slices in a large bowl. Add mixture of water, lemon juice, and Sucaryl; stir again. Put in a 6- by 10-inch baking dish that has been sprayed with PAM. After sprinkling with topping (topping recipe follows), bake in 350-degree oven for 45 minutes.

Topping for Deep-Dish Apple Pie

    1   cup grated Cheddar Cheese
    ³/₄   cup Biscuit Mix
    1   tablespoon powdered Sucaryl

Combine all ingredients and sprinkle over apple mixture that's been placed in baking dish.

One serving (pie with topping) equals ¹/₂ Milk Exchange, 1 Fruit Exchange, 1 Fat Exchange.

- - - - - - - - - -

Exchanges for one serving of the entire menu equal ¹/₂ Milk, 1 A Vegetable, 1 Fruit, 1 Bread, 3 Meat, 3 Fat.

* * * * *

WEEKEND LUNCHES

A planned weekend lunch can be a happy experience. It's a temptation just to snack from the refrigerator to save time; but this is not recommended. Organize your lunch ahead of time and you will love the results.

If the weather is nice, try eating on the porch or in the garden. If it is snowy and blustery, eat in front of the fire with a TV tray for a table, and feel cozy. Food always tastes better when a little atmosphere is added, and this can be created right in your own home. Make an occasion out of any meal that you plan and your whole life will become more interesting.

Menus and Recipes for Two

Border Tostado

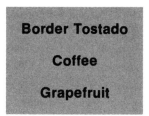

Border Tostado

Coffee

Grapefruit

Border Tostado (2 servings — 1 tostado each)

2   corn Tortillas (about 6 inches in diameter)
1/2   cup grated Monterrey Jack Cheese
1   ounce canned whole Green Chili (seeded and chopped)
2   teaspoons minced Onion
1/8   teaspoon ground Cumin
1/8   teaspoon Salt
1/4   cup shredded Lettuce

Bake tortillas on cookie sheet in 300-degree oven until crisp (about 45 minutes), watching carefully to prevent burning. These may be baked the day before using.

Mix grated cheese with cumin, chili, and onion. Spread half the mixture on each tortilla. Broil until cheese is melted. Top with shredded lettuce and serve.

One serving equals 1 Bread Exchange, 1 Meat Exchange.

Grapefruit (2 servings — ¹/₂ grapefruit each)

Remove seeds and loosen sections of grapefruit. A blueberry or strawberry may be used as a garnish.
One serving equals 1 Fruit Exchange.

- - - - - - - - - -

Exchanges for one serving of the entire menu equal 1 Fruit, 1 Bread, 1 Meat.

* * * * *

Overnight Soufflé

Overnight Soufflé

Melon in Season   **Coffee or Tea**

Overnight Soufflé (2 servings – 1 sandwich each)

4	thin slices Bread
4	ounces sharp Cheddar Cheese, grated
1	cup Milk
1	Egg, beaten
2	teaspoons grated Onion

Make two sandwiches of bread, cheese, and onion, reserving about 2 teaspoons of grated cheese. Put sandwiches in a casserole that has been sprayed with PAM, and sprinkle remaining cheese on top. Combine milk and egg, and pour this over sandwiches. Cover and refrigerate over night. When ready to serve, bake in 350-degree oven for 30 minutes.

One serving equals ½ Milk Exchange, 1½ Bread Exchanges, 2½ Meat Exchanges.

Melon in Season (2 servings – 1 cup each)

Melons that may be used are watermelon, cantaloupe, honeydew melon, and muskmelon. Cut melon in sections that would yield about 1 cup. Serve cold.

One serving equals 1 Fruit Exchange.

- - - - - - - - - -

Exchanges for one serving of the entire menu equal ½ Milk, 1 Fruit, 1½ Bread, 2½ Meat.

* * * * *

Tomato Stuffed with Egg Salad

Tomato Stuffed with Egg Salad

Dill Pickle Fingers

Hot Roll

Tomato Stuffed with Egg Salad (2 servings — 1 tomato each)

2	medium-sized Tomatoes
2	hard-boiled Eggs
2	teaspoons Vinegar
2	tablespoons Mayonnaise
$1/8$	teaspoon Dill Weed

Salt and Pepper
2   Lettuce Leaves

Dice eggs and mix with mayonnaise, vinegar, dill weed, salt, and pepper. Remove thin slice from top of both tomatoes, then cut each almost through into quarters and place on a lettuce leaf. After spreading the tomatoes apart slightly, put half of the filling on each.

One serving equals 1 A Vegetable Exchange, 1 Meat Exchange, 3 Fat Exchanges.

Dill Pickle Fingers (2 servings — $1/2$ pickle each)

1   large Dill Pickle, quartered lengthwise.

One serving equals Zero Exchange.

Hot Roll (2 servings — 1 roll each)

Split 2 small rolls and toast lightly. Serve hot.
One serving equals 1 Bread Exchange.

- - - - - - - - - -

Exchanges for one serving of the entire menu equal 1 A Vegetable, 1 Bread, 1 Meat, 3 Fat.

* * * * *

Pizza

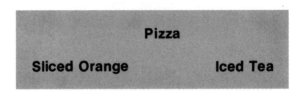

Pizza

Sliced Orange   **Iced Tea**

Pizza (2 servings — 2 half muffins each)

2   *English Muffins (at room temperature)*
3   *ounces ground Beef*
2   *ounces Mozzarelli Cheese*
4   *tablespoons Tomato Paste*
1   *tablespoon Water*
1/2 *teaspoon Oregano*
1   *pinch of Salt*

Cook beef in skillet until lightly browned. Split muffins in half and flatten each half with rolling pin, being careful not to split the edges. Mix tomato paste and water, add oregano and salt, and spread on muffin halves. Sprinkle with cooked meat and top with slices of cheese. Heat in 450-degree oven until cheese melts (about 8 minutes).
One serving equals 2 Bread Exchanges, 2 Meat Exchanges.

Sliced Orange (2 servings — 1 orange each)

Peel and slice 2 medium-sized oranges.
One serving equals 2 Fruit Exchanges.

- - - - - - - - - -

Exchanges for one serving of the entire menu equal 2 Fruit, 2 Bread, 2 Meat.

* * * * *

Hamburger on Bun

Milk

Hamburger on a Bun

Horseradish   Mustard

Onion Slices

Lettuce   Dill Pickle

Apple

Milk (2 servings — ¹/₂ pint each)

One serving equals 1 Milk Exchange.

Hamburger on a Bun (2 servings — 1 hamburger each)

6   *ounces lean ground Beef*
2   *small Hamburger Buns*
¹/₂ *Onion, sliced thin*
1   *Lettuce Leaf, shredded*
1   *Dill Pickle, sliced thin*
Cream Horseradish
Mustard
Salt and Pepper

Shape ground meat into two patties of equal size. Prepare onion, dill pickle, and lettuce. Split hamburger buns. Broil meat patties until brown on each side. Serve meat on bun, offering the onion, lettuce, pickle, and condiments on a side tray.

One serving equals ¹/₂ A Vegetable Exchange, 2 Bread Exchanges, 2 Meat Exchanges.

Apple (2 servings — 1 apple each)

One small apple equals 1 Fruit Exchange.

- - - - - - - - - -

Exchanges for one serving of the entire menu equal 1 Milk, ¹/₂ A Vegetable, 1 Fruit, 2 Bread, 2 Meat.

* * * * *

BRIDGE LUNCHEONS

Cards and calories share equal honors in conversation when the gals gather at a bridge luncheon. Whether a diabetic or not, aren't most of your lady friends weight conscious? The plump ones are interested in cutting down, and the thin ones are interested in keeping down. They will love coming to your home for a bridge luncheon when any of the following menus are served. The diabetic won't have to be concerned about the fare and the nondiabetic won't realize that it is a diet luncheon that she is eating.

Menus and Recipes for Four

Stuffed Eggplant

Stuffed Eggplant

Carrot Curls

Toasted Triangles

Meringues with Jam and Topping

Tea or Coffee

Stuffed Eggplant (4 servings — ¹/₂ eggplant each)

2	small Eggplants
1	cup cooked Crab Meat
2	cups Tomatoes
¹/₂	Green Pepper, diced
¹/₂	cup dry Bread Crumbs
1	medium-sized Onion, diced
¹/₈	teaspoon Rosemary
¹/₂	teaspoon Sweet Basil

Salt and Pepper

Split eggplants in half lengthwise. Boil in enough salted water to cover, until tender, about 5 minutes (until they can be pierced with a fork). Drain well. Scoop insides from eggplants, leaving the shells intact. Dice the insides and mix with remaining ingredients. Place mixture in the eggplant shells and bake in 300-degree oven for 30 minutes. Serve hot.

One serving equals 2 A Vegetable Exchanges, ¹/₂ Bread Exchange, 1 Meat Exchange.

Carrot Curls (4 servings — 3 to 4 curls each)

3   large Carrots, scraped.

Cut the carrots into very thin strips lengthwise with a vegetable peeler. (This may take a little practice, but is worth it.) Roll and secure each strip with a toothpick, forming curls. Store the carrot curls in refrigerator in ice water. When ready to serve remove the toothpicks.
One serving equals ¹/₂ B Vegetable Exchange.

Toasted Triangles (4 servings — 1 triangle each)

4   thin slices Bread
4   teaspoons Margarine

Spread each bread slice with 1 teaspoon margarine. Put butter sides together and cut diagonally, making triangles. Bake in 400-degree oven until slightly toasted (about 5 minutes). Serve hot.
One serving equals ³/₄ Bread Exchange, 1 Fat Exchange.

Meringues with Jam and Topping
(4 servings — 1 meringue each)

2   Egg Whites
¹/₄   cup dry Skim Milk
1¹/₃ teaspoons liquid Sucaryl
¹/₄   teaspoon Vanilla Flavoring

Beat egg whites until they peak, then add vanilla flavoring and Sucaryl and mix well. Add powdered milk slowly, beating constantly until the batter is smooth. Spray cookie sheet with PAM and divide the mixture into four tall piles on the cookie sheet. With a spoon, shape each pile into a cup by hollowing out the center. Bake in preheated 275-degree oven for 40 minutes.

Jam for Meringues (4 servings — ¹/₄ cup each)

> 2   cups *Fruit (peaches, plums, or berries)*
> 1   teaspoon *Lemon Juice*
> ¹/₄   cup *Water*
> 2   teaspoons *Cornstarch*
> 1   teaspoon *liquid Sucaryl*

Cook fruit over slow heat for 10 minutes. (Be sure that you have enough water; some fruits need more than others.) Add lemon juice and mix well.

Mix cornstarch with water and cook until it is clear (about 2 minutes), then cool. Combine both mixtures and add Sucaryl. Stir well and refrigerate.

Topping for Meringues (4 servings — 2 tablespoons each)

Use recipe for Jane's Topping given in Part IV (see Index), but use one-fourth of the quantities listed.

Each serving (1 meringue, ¹/₄ cup of jam, and 2 tablespoons of topping) equals ¹/₃ Skim Milk Exchange, 1 Fruit Exchange.

- - - - - - - - - -

Exchanges for one serving of the entire menu equal ¹/₃ Skim Milk, 2 A Vegetable, ¹/₂ B Vegetable, 1 Fruit, 1¹/₄ Bread, 1 Meat, 1 Fat.

* * * * *

Chicken Salad

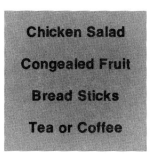

Chicken Salad

Congealed Fruit

Bread Sticks

Tea or Coffee

Chicken Salad (4 servings — 1¹/₄ cups each)

8   *ounces cooked Chicken or Turkey*
1   *cup chopped Celery*
2   *Scallions, chopped fine*
4   *tablespoons Mayonnaise*
1   *tablespoon Lemon Juice*
4   *Lettuce Leaves*
Salt and Pepper

Cube meat and add remaining ingredients except lettuce. The flavor is enhanced if the salad is made the day before and stored in refrigerator. Serve on lettuce leaf.

One serving equals 1 A Vegetable Exchange, 2 Meat Exchanges, 3 Fat Exchanges.

Congealed Fruit (4 servings — ¹/₂ cup each)

1   *package Raspberry D-Zerta*
2   *cups water-packed Pears, drained and diced*
4   *Lettuce Leaves*

Prepare D-Zerta according to directions on package. When cool, add pears and pour into four individual molds. Serve on lettuce leaf.

One serving equals 1 Fruit Exchange.

Bread Sticks (4 servings—2 sticks each)

   8   *Bread Sticks (commercial size)*

One serving equals ½ Bread Exchange.

- - - - - - - - - -

Exchanges for one serving of the entire menu equal 1 A Vegetable, 1 Fruit, ½ Bread, 2 Meat, 3 Fat.

* * * * *

Casino Sandwich

Orange-Lime Cooler

Casino Sandwich

Spinach and Egg Salad

Broiled Peach Half

Hot Tea

Orange-Lime Cooler (4 servings — $1/2$ cup each)

1	cup Lime Juice
1	cup Orange Juice
$1/4$	teaspoon liquid Sucaryl
$1/4$	teaspoon Angostura Bitters

Combine all ingredients and pour over crushed ice in glasses. One serving equals 1 Fruit Exchange.

Casino Sandwich (4 servings — $1/2$ sandwich each)

4	thin slices Bread
4	ounces Ham, sliced very thin
4	ounces Monterrey Jack Cheese, grated
1	Egg
2	tablespoons Milk
4	teaspoons Salad Oil

Make sandwiches with ham, cheese, and bread. Beat egg with milk. Dip each sandwich in egg mixture. Heat oil in skillet and toast each sandwich on both sides. Cut each sandwich into quarters for serving.

One serving equals ¾ Bread Exchange, 2 Meat Exchanges, 1 Fat Exchange.

Spinach and Egg Salad (4 servings—1 cup each)

4	cups fresh Spinach
1	cup imitation Sour Cream
2	tablespoons Vinegar
2	hard-boiled Eggs, chopped
¼	Onion, chopped fine

Wash spinach carefully and cut off stems. Drain well and tear into bite-size pieces, removing veins that are tough. Wrap in paper towels and refrigerate to crisp. Mix vinegar and sour cream. When ready to serve, toss all ingredients together.

One serving equals 1 A Vegetable Exchange, ½ Milk Exchange, 1 Fat Exchange.

Broiled Peach Halves (4 servings—½ peach each)

4	water-packed canned Peach Halves
2	teaspoons Brown-Sugar Substitute

Put peach halves in broiling pan and sprinkle with sugar substitute. Broil until bubbly. Serve hot.

One serving equals 1 Fruit Exchange.

- - - - - - - - - -

Exchanges for one serving of the entire menu equal ½ Milk, 1 A Vegetable, 2 Fruit, ¾ Bread, 2 Meat, 2 Fat.

* * * * *

Seafood Supreme

Seafood Supreme

Broiled Tomato with Cheese

Marinated Asparagus

Hot Rolls with Margarine

Seafood Supreme
(4 servings — 3 ounces fish and 1 shrimp each)

12   ounces Flounder Fillets (4 Fillets sliced thin)
4   large raw Shrimp, peeled
4   teaspoons Margarine, softened
3/4   cup dry White Wine
Salt and Pepper

Spread margarine over fillets (1 teaspoon per fillet), then sprinkle them with salt and pepper. Roll each fillet around 1 shrimp, secure with a toothpick, and place in a baking dish that has been sprayed with PAM. Pour wine over the fillet-shrimp rings and bake them in 450-degree oven for 20 minutes. Baste two or three times while cooking. Do not overcook. Serve hot.
One serving equals 2 Meat Exchanges, 1 Fat Exchange.

Broiled Tomato with Cheese (4 servings — 1 tomato each)

4   medium-sized Tomatoes
2   tablespoons grated Parmesan Cheese
1   teaspoon chopped Chives
1/2   teaspoon Oregano
Salt and Pepper

Cut a thin slice off the top of each tomato. Partially quarter each tomato and spread open. Sprinkle with herbs, salt, and pepper. Top with cheese. Broil until cheese is bubbly. Serve hot.

One serving equals 1 A Vegetable Exchange.

Marinated Asparagus* (4 servings—6 to 8 spears each)

1	*1-pound can Asparagus Spears*
	Juice of ½ Lemon
½	*cup Cider Vinegar*
3	*teaspoons liquid Sucaryl*
1	*teaspoon Salt*
1	*teaspoon Seasoned Pepper*

Drain asparagus, retaining the juice. Mix all other ingredients with asparagus juice, pour over asparagus in a suitable dish. Cover and refrigerate over night. (This will keep for 2 weeks.) Serve cold.

One serving equals 1 A Vegetable Exchange.

Hot Rolls with Margarine (4 servings—1 roll each)

4	*Rolls, 2 inches in diameter*
4	*teaspoons Margarine*

Put 1 teaspoon margarine on each roll. Heat rolls thoroughly in hot oven. Serve Hot.

One serving equals 1 Bread Exchange, 1 Fat Exchange.

- - - - - - - - - -

Exchanges for one serving of the entire menu equal 2 A Vegetable, 1 Bread, 2 Meat, 2 Fat.

* * * * *

*Prepare the Marinated Asparagus the day before serving.

Ham Salad on Lettuce

Ham Salad on Lettuce

Sliced Orange

Toasted English Muffin

Tea or Coffee or Diet Drinks

Ham Salad on Lettuce (4 servings — $1/2$ cup each)

8	ounces lean boiled or canned Ham
4	teaspoons Mayonnaise
2	tablespoons Lemon Juice
1	teaspoon grated Onion
2	tablespoons minced Celery
4	Lettuce leaves

Chop ham and mix with remaining ingredients. Serve each portion on a lettuce leaf.

One serving equals 1 A Vegetable Exchange, 2 Meat Exchanges, 1 Fat Exchange.

Sliced Orange (4 servings — 1 orange each)

4	medium-sized Navel Oranges

Peel each orange, slice thin, and arrange on a plate with ham salad.

One serving equals 2 Fruit Exchanges.

Toasted Muffins (4 servings — ¹/₂ muffin each)

2   *English muffins*

Split the muffins and toast them. Serve hot.
One serving equals 1 Bread Exchange.

- - - - - - - - - -

Exchanges for one serving of the entire menu equal 1 A Vegetable, 2 Fruit, 1 Bread, 2 Meat, 1 Fat.

* * * * *

BUFFETS

A buffet provides a popular approach for group entertaining, especially for family members and/or guests having diet restrictions. When more than one entree is indicated the food can be portioned in half servings so that a choice can be made: two half portions of one entree, or a half portion of each.

Table decorations will aid in making a buffet distinctive. A special theme apropos of the occasion (e.g., a birthday, anniversary, holiday) or the season can be employed. For a St. Patrick's Day party, holders or pots for jonquils or other early spring flowers can be made from Irish potatoes. Paint the potatoes bright green and brush their eyes with gold. Scoop out the insides, retaining enough of the scooped potato to act as a holder for the flowers. For a fall party, decorative gourds can be scooped out and used as containers for button marigolds or dwarf chrysanthemums.

Menus and Recipes for Ten

Rib Eye Roast

Spiced Apple Drink

Rib Eye Roast   **Horseradish Sauce**

Celery Stuffed with Pimiento Cheese

Marinated Green Beans

Scalloped Rice

Angel Food Cake* with Apricot Jam

Spiced Apple Drink (10 servings — 1 cup each)

    8   cans diet Apple Drink
    2   sticks Cinnamon
    3   whole Cloves
    1/3 cup Water

Boil the stick cinnamon and cloves in water for about 5 minutes. Cool. When ready to serve, pour thoroughly chilled apple drink in a pitcher and add the essence of cinnamon-clove.
One serving equals Zero Exchange.

*Contains small amount of sugar.

Rib Eye Roast (10 servings — 3 ounces each)

1	*Rib Eye Roast (5 pounds)*
$1/4$	*cup Madeira Wine*
$1/4$	*teaspoon Dry Mustard*
$1/4$	*teaspoon powdered Mushrooms*
1	*teaspoon Soy Sauce*
$2^2/3$	*tablespoons Margarine*
$1/2$	*teaspoon Salt*
$1/2$	*teaspoon coarse ground Pepper*

Combine wine and seasonings; marinate meat in this mixture over night in refrigerator, or at least $2^1/2$ hours at room temperature, turning occasionally. Place meat in an uncovered roasting pan in a cold oven; cook at 300 degrees for 2 hours, basting every 15 minutes with remaining marinade to which has been added the melted margarine.

One serving equals 3 Meat Exchanges, 1 Fat Exchange.

Horseradish Sauce (10 servings — $1/2$ tablespoons each)

8	*tablespoons Prepared Horseradish*
1	*cup Sour Cream*

Mix ingredients thoroughly. Serve cold.
One serving equals 1 Fat Exchange.

Celery Stuffed with Pimiento Cheese
(10 servings — 3 pieces each)

5	*ounces Cream Cheese*
10	*ribs Celery*
2	*Pimientos, chopped*
2	*tablespoons Milk*

Salt and Pepper

Mix milk, cheese, pimientos, and salt and pepper. Cut each rib of celery into three pieces and stuff with cheese mixture.
One serving equals 1 A Vegetable Exchange, 1 Fat Exchange.

Marinated Green Beans (10 servings — ¹/₂ cup each)

2   cans (16 ounces each) whole Green Beans
1   cup Cider Vinegar
4   teaspoons liquid Sucaryl
2   teaspoons Salt
1   teaspoon Seasoned Pepper

Drain beans, reserving juice; place beans in a casserole. Combine remaining ingredients and pour over the beans. If more liquid is needed to cover beans, use the reserved juice. Cover and refrigerate over night.
One serving equals 1 A Vegetable Exchange.

Scalloped Rice (10 servings — ¹/₂ cup each)

5   cups cooked Rice
1¹/₂ tablespoons Flour
1¹/₂ teaspoons Salt
1   cup chopped Green Onion
²/₃ cup chopped Parsley
2¹/₂ cups Light Cream

Mix all ingredients except cream and place in casserole that has been sprayed with PAM. Pour cream over all. Bake uncovered in 350-degree oven for 30 minutes, or until set.
One serving equals 1 Bread Exchange, 1¹/₂ Fat Exchanges.

Angel Food Cake* (12 servings)

1	cup plus 2 tablespoons Flour
$^1/_2$	cup Sugar
12	Egg Whites
$^1/_8$	teaspoon Salt
1	teaspoon Cream of Tartar
1	tablespoon liquid Sucaryl
1	teaspoon Vanilla Flavoring
$^1/_2$	teaspoon Almond Flavoring

Sift flour, sugar, and salt together several times. Beat egg whites until frothy and add cream of tartar. Continue beating until whites are stiff but not dry. Add Sucaryl and flavorings. Fold dry ingredients into egg whites rapidly but carefully. Pour into large ungreased angel food pan and bake in 325-degree oven about 1 hour, or until cake shrinks from side of pan. Remove from oven and turn upside down to cool.

COMMENT: After much experimenting it was found that it was necessary to use a small amount of sugar for the cake to hold up as "angel food."

One serving equals 1 Bread Exchange.

Apricot Jam for Angel Food Cake (10 servings — $^1/_2$ cup each)

80	halves dried Apricots, quartered
2	tablespoons Lemon Juice
4	teaspoons Gelatin
1	tablespoon Water
1	teaspoon Vanilla Flavoring
$^1/_2$	teaspoon Almond Flavoring
1	tablespoon liquid Sucaryl

*Contains small amount of sugar.

After soaking the dried apricots over night in just enough cold water to cover them, add lemon juice and cook over low heat for about 30 minutes, being careful that they do not scorch. Remove from heat. Soften gelatin in water, add to hot fruit, and stir. Cool. Add flavorings and Sucaryl. Taste and add more Sucaryl if desired.

One serving equals 1 Fruit Exchange.

- - - - - - - - - -

Exchanges for one serving of the entire menu equal 2 A Vegetable, 1 Fruit, 2 Bread, 3 Meat, 4¹/₂ Fat.

* * * * *

Chicken Casserole—King Ranch Style

Gazpacho

Chicken Casserole—King Ranch Style

Relish Tray

Asparagus with Lemon Butter

Pineapple Hawaiian

Gazpacho (10 servings — ²/₃ cup each)

3	cups Tomato Juice
2	Cucumbers, peeled
2	large fresh Tomatoes
1	large Green Pepper
3	tablespoons Parsley, chopped fine
¹/₄	cup Red Wine Vinegar
¹/₂	cup chopped Celery
¹/₂	teaspoon Garlic Powder
1	teaspoon Salt
¹/₄	teaspoon Tabasco Sauce
2	tablespoons chopped Chives

Put all ingredients except chives in blender. Mix at medium speed until all ingredients are pulverized. Chill. Serve in cups, with chopped chives sprinkled on top.

One serving equals 2 A Vegetable Exchanges.

Chicken Casserole—King Ranch Style
(10 servings — ³/₄ cup each)

2	pounds cooked Chicken
1	can Condensed Cream of Mushroom Soup
1½	cups Chicken Broth
8	ounces Velveeta Cheese
1	can Tomatoes and Green Chiles
10	corn Tortillas
½	small Onion

Chop chicken in bite-size pieces after removing skin. Cook chopped onion in half a cup of chicken broth until onion is clear. Add rest of broth, the tomatoes and chiles, and cream of mushroom soup.

Dip the tortillas, one at a time, in the soupy mixture to soften, then put a thin layer of the softened tortillas in a casserole. Add a layer of chicken with some of the soupy mixture and a layer of cheese. Add another thin layer of softened tortillas, a layer of chicken with the soupy mixture, and a layer of cheese. If is it necessary to make a series of three layers, instead of two, let the top layer be cheese. Bake in 350-degree over for 30 minutes, or until bubbles appear in the middle.

This casserole may be prepared for baking several days before it is planned to be served and kept in the refrigerator until time to bake it.

One serving equals 1 Bread Exchange, 4 Meat Exchanges, ½ Fat Exchange.

Relish Tray (10 servings)

2	Zucchini
3	Carrots
2	bunches Radishes
2	bunches Green Onions

Cut unpeeled zucchini into thin slices. Cut carrots into strips about 2¹/₂ inches long and ¹/₄ inch wide. Prepare radishes and green onions. Arrange on relish tray.
One serving equals 1 A Vegetable Exchange.

Asparagus with Lemon Butter (10 servings — 3 ounces each)

3   *10-ounce packages frozen Asparagus Spears*
4   *tablespoons Lemon Juice*
¹/₂   *teaspoon Butter Flavoring*

Cook asparagus according to directions on package. Do not overcook. Drain and add lemon juice to which has been added the butter flavoring. Serve hot.
One serving equals 1 A Vegetable Exchange.

Pineapple Hawaiian (10 servings — ¹/₄ pineapple each)

3   *small fresh Pineapples*
10   *rounded tablespoons toasted Coconut*
Granulated Sucaryl

Cut pineapples in quarters lengthwise, cutting through stems at top. With a small knife, cut down both sides of each section to remove the edible pulp. Cut the hard center out of each piece and discard it. Cut pulp into bite-size pieces and sprinkle with Sucaryl if desired. Mix with coconut and return to shells to serve. Instead of the coconut a few drops of Angostura Bitters or a few drops of mint flavoring may be substituted.
Strawberries or blueberries complement pineapple and may be used as a garnish.
One serving equals 1 Fruit Exchange.

- - - - - - - - - -

Exchanges for one serving of the entire menu equal 4 A Vegetable, 1 Fruit, 1 Bread, 4 Meat, ¹/₂ Fat.

* * * * *

Meat Loaf-Shrimp Salad

Meat Loaf

Shrimp Salad

Broccoli and Rice Casserole

Carrot and Celery Sticks

Marinated Beet and Onion Rings

Fresh Fruit in Season

Meat Loaf (10 servings—3 ounces each)

2¹/₂ pounds lean ground Beef
³/₄   cup Quick-Cooking Oatmeal
1¹/₂ cups Tomato Juice
1   Egg, slightly beaten
¹/₂   cup finely chopped Onion
1   teaspoon Salt
1   teaspoon Pepper

Combine all ingredients. Shape into a loaf and put in a baking dish or pan. Bake in 350-degree oven for 1¹/₄ hours. Cool slightly, then divide into 10 equal slices.

One serving equals ¹/₄ Bread Exchange, 3 Meat Exchanges.

Shrimp Salad (10 servings — ¹/₂ cup each)

50 medium-sized Shrimp, cooked and peeled
1 cup Celery, chopped
3 hard-boiled Eggs, chopped
1¹/₂ cups minced unsweetened Dill Pickles
1¹/₄ cups Dressing (recipe follows)
1 tablespoon Lemon Juice
2 tablespoons Capers (optional)
Salt and Pepper
10 Lettuce Leaves

Mix all ingredients except lettuce thoroughly but gently. Cover and set in refrigerator an hour or so to blend flavors. Serve on lettuce leaves.

Dressing for Shrimp Salad (10 servings — 1 tablespoon each)

1¹/₂ teaspoons Gelatin
2 tablespoons Water
1 cup Buttermilk
2 tablespoons Salad Oil
Juice of 3 Lemons
1 tablespoon Worcestershire Sauce
1 teaspoon Salt
1 teaspoon Dry Mustard

Put water in small pan and sprinkle gelatin on top. When gelatin has softened, turn heat on low and stir until gelatin has dissolved. Pour part of buttermilk into gelatin and stir well. Remove from heat. After the mixture has jelled, place it in blender with remaining ingredients and blend until smooth. This dressing will keep well in the refrigerator and may be made several days in advance of its use.

One serving (shrimp mixture and dressing) equals 1 Meat Exchange, ¹/₂ Fat Exchange.

Broccoli and Rice Casserole (10 servings — 1 cup each)

2	10-ounce packages frozen chopped Broccoli
4	teaspoons Margarine
2	medium-sized Onions, chopped
1¹/₂	cups uncooked Rice
2	cans Condensed Cream of Mushroom Soup
16	ounces Velveeta Cheese
1	cup low-fat Milk

Salt and Pepper

Sauté onion and broccoli slowly in margarine. Add mushroom soup. Cook rice as directed on package, and while it is still hot add the cheese. When cheese is melted, add milk and the broccoli mixture. Bake in 350-degree oven for 30 minutes. Serve hot.

One serving equals 1 A Vegetable Exchange, 1 Bread Exchange, 2 Meat Exchanges, ¹/₂ Fat Exchange.

Carrot and Celery Sticks (10 servings)

5	medium-sized Carrots
5	ribs Celery

Clean carrots and celery and cut into strips. Store in refrigerator hydrator several hours to crisp.

One serving equals ¹/₂ A Vegetable Exchange, ¹/₂ B Vegetable Exchange.

Marinated Beet and Onion Rings (10 servings — ¹/₂ cup each)

4	cups cooked sliced Beets
1	large White Onion, sliced very thin
¹/₂	cup Vinegar
¹/₄	cup granulated Sucaryl

Juice of 1 Lemon
Salt

Drain beets, reserving juice. Mix onion and beets in casserole. Combine remaining ingredients and pour them over vegetables. If there is not sufficient juice to cover, add some of reserved beet juice. Cover and refrigerate over night.

One serving equals 1 B Vegetable Exchange.

Fresh Fruits in Season (10 servings — 1 fruit exchange each)

The following fruit portions contain 1 Fruit Exchange each. Select 10 portions and arrange on platter or chop plate.

1	*2-inch Apple*
2	*medium-sized Apricots*
$1/2$	*small Banana*
$2/3$	*cup Blueberries*
1	*cup Strawberries*
$1/2$	*small Cantaloupe*
$1/2$	*small Grapefruit*
12	*Grapes*
1	*small Orange*
1	*medium-sized Peach*
$1/2$	*cup unsweetened Pineapple*
1	*large Tangerine*

- - - - - - - - - -

Exchanges for one serving of the entire menu equal 1½ A Vegetable, 1½ B Vegetable, 1 Fruit, 1¼ Bread, 6 Meat, 1 Fat.

* * * * *

Holiday Turkey

Holiday Turkey

Dressing and Gravy

Cranberry Chutney   **Green Beans**

Grapefruit and Orange Salad

Scotch Coffee

Holiday Turkey (servings should be 3 ounces each)

1   *large Turkey (12 to 15 pounds)*
4   *tablespoons Flour*
Salt and Pepper

When turkey is defrosted (if frozen), remove giblets and neck from body cavity. Wash giblets, cover with water, and simmer until tender (about 2 hours).

Rinse outside and inside of turkey with cold water. Rub salt and pepper into cavity and on outside of turkey. Place turkey in shallow pan; cover breast area with aluminum foil. Roast in 300-degree oven 20 minutes per pound. Remove foil for the last hour to brown the bird, basting several times with its own juice.

Gravy

When giblets and neck are cool, remove them from the water in which they were cooked. Chop giblets and neck meat then return them to the cooking water. Carefully skim the grease from the pan in which the turkey was roasted. Add the broth containing the giblets and neck meat to the drippings left in the roasting pan. Estimate amount of liquid, and add water if necessary to make 4 cups. Mix flour with a little water, and stir into heated giblet broth and drippings. Cook until thickened. Salt and pepper to taste.

One 3-ounce serving of turkey with 2 ounces of gravy equals 3 Meat Exchanges, 2 Fat Exchanges.

Dressing (10 servings — ²/₃ cup each)

2	medium-sized Onions, chopped
1	cup chopped Celery
6	slices White Bread, dried and crumbled
6	1¹/₂-inch cubes Cornbread, crumbled
2	teaspoons powdered Sage
2	Eggs, beaten
2	cups Milk

Salt and Pepper

Cook onion and celery in small amount of water for about 10 minutes. Mix all ingredients together, using only enough milk to moisten (all the milk may not be required). Mixture should be moist but not soupy. Bake in casserole in 325-degree oven for 40 minutes.

One serving equals 1¹/₂ Bread Exchanges, ¹/₂ Fat Exchange.

Cranberry Chutney (10 servings — ⁵/₈ cup each)

1	can (16 ounces) peeled Tomatoes, including liquid
4	cups fresh Cranberries
³/₄	cup Raisins
³/₄	cup granulated Sucaryl
1	clove Garlic, minced
¹/₂	teaspoon Cinnamon
¹/₄	teaspoon Ginger
1	teaspoon Salt

Chop or grind raisins, then mix all ingredients except Sucaryl. Bring to a boil, stirring frequently. Simmer for 15 minutes, then add Sucaryl. Refrigerate several days to blend flavors.

One serving equals 1 Fruit Exchange.

Green Beans (10 servings — 1/2 cup each)

3	*10-ounce packages frozen Green Beans*
1/2	*teaspoon Butter Flavoring*

Cook beans according to directions on package; pour off water, reserving 2 tablespoons. Combine butter flavoring with reserved water and pour over beans. Serve hot.

One serving equals 1 A Vegetable Exchange.

Grapefruit and Orange Salad (10 servings — 2/3 cup each)

2	*tablespoons Gelatin*
1/2	*cup cold Water*
1	*cup boiling Water*
3/4	*teaspoon liquid Sucaryl*
3	*cups fresh Grapefruit Sections, cut into pieces*
2	*cups fresh Orange Sections, cut into pieces*

Sprinkle gelatin over cold water. When clear, add boiling water and stir until gelatin is dissolved. Cool and add Sucaryl. Refrigerate until mixture jells. Stir in the fruit and put in molds (10 individual or 1 large).

One serving equals 1 Fruit Exchange.

Scotch Coffee (10 servings — 2/3 cup each)

6	*cups very strong Coffee*
1 1/2	*teaspoons liquid Sucaryl*
2	*teaspoons Brandy Flavoring*
10	*tablespoons Whipped Cream*

Blend coffee, brandy flavoring, and Sucaryl. Pour into heated parfait glasses, top each with 1 tablespoon whipped cream.

One serving equals 1 Fat Exchange.

- - - - - - - - - -

Exchanges for one serving of the entire menu equal 1 A Vegetable, 2 Fruit, 1½ Bread, 3 Meat, 3½ Fat.

* * * * *

Chicken a la King on Toast Triangles - Fish Fillet in Sauterne

Chicken a la King on Toast Triangles

Fish Fillet in Sauterne

Eggplant Italian

Astronomical Fruit with Jane's Topping

Strawberry Cream Pie

Chicken a la King on Toast Triangles
(10 servings — 1/2 cup each)

1¹/₂	pounds cooked Chicken, diced
10	tablespoons Margarine
10	tablespoons Flour
3³/₄	cups Skim Milk
1	teaspoon Salt
2	teaspoons grated Onion
1	teaspoon Worcestershire Sauce
¹/₄	teaspoon Tabasco Sauce
3	tablespoons minced Parsley
2	tablespoons chopped Pimiento
	Paprika (optional)
10	Toast Triangles, ¹/₄ slice of Bread for each

Melt margarine, add flour, and gradually add milk, stirring constantly. Cook until thickened. Add seasonings, pimiento, parsley, and chicken. When thoroughly heated, remove from stove and serve on toast triangles. Sprinkle with paprika.

One serving equals ½ Bread Exchange, 2 Meat Exchanges, 2 Fat Exchanges.

Fish Fillet in Sauterne (10 servings — 2 ounces each)

    2½   pounds frozen Fish Fillets
    1   small clove Garlic, crushed
    ¼   teaspoon Thyme
    2   cups Sauterne Wine
    3   tablespoons Margarine
    2   tablespoons Capers
    1   Bay Leaf
    Salt and Pepper

Place thawed fish fillets in flat baking dish, season with salt and pepper. Mix other ingredients and pour over fish. Dot with margarine. Cover and bake in 325-degree oven for 30 minutes, or until fish flakes when pierced with a fork. Do not overcook.

One serving equals 2 Meat Exchanges, 1 Fat Exchange.

Eggplant Italian (10 servings — 1 slice each)

    2   large Eggplants
    1¼   cups Marinara Sauce (recipe follows)
    10   tablespoons grated Italian Cheese
    1   teaspoon Oregano

Cut unpeeled eggplants into ¾-inch slices. Sprinkle with salt and let stand 30 minutes; then wipe dry with paper towels. Sear eggplant in skillet that has been sprayed with PAM, being careful not to tear slices. Mix marinara sauce with oregano. Arrange eggplant slices in large, flat casserole, and put 2 table-spoons sauce over each slice. Top with 1 tablespoon grated cheese. Bake in 350-degree oven for 30 minutes.

Marinara Sauce

4	ounces Tomato Paste
1	cup Water
1	tablespoon Salt
1	clove Garlic, mashed
1¹/₂	teaspoons Oregano
¹/₂	teaspoon Sweet Basil
¹/₄	teaspoon Rosemary
1	Bay Leaf

Combine all ingredients and simmer for 20 minutes. Remove bay leaf. Yields about 1¹/₂ cups.

One serving (eggplant with sauce) equals 1 A Vegetable Exchange, ¹/₂ Fat Exchange.

Astronomical Fruit (10 servings — ¹/₂ cup each)

1	cup Bananas, mashed
1¹/₂	cups diced unsweetened Pineapple
1	cup unsweetened Strawberries
1	cup Pears, fresh or water-packed
1	large unpeeled Apple, diced
10	tablespoons Jane's Topping*

Mix all ingredients (fruits and topping) thoroughly.
One serving equals 1 Fruit Exchange.

*Use recipe for Jane's Topping given in Part IV (see Index), but cut to one-third the quantities designated.

Strawberry Cream Pie (10 servings — ¹/₅ pie each)

Crust

> 6 *Egg Whites*
> ³/₄ *cup powdered Milk*
> 4 *teaspoons liquid Sucaryl*
> ¹/₂ *teaspoon Vanilla Flavoring*
> ¹/₈ *teaspoon Almond Flavoring*

Beat egg whites until peaks form. Add 4 teaspoons liquid Sucaryl and flavorings. Add powdered milk gradually, while beating, until there is a smooth paste. Spread over bottoms and up the edges of two Pyrex pie pans that have been sprayed with PAM. Bake in preheated 275-degree oven for 30 minutes. Cool.

Filling

> 6 *Egg Yolks*
> ²/₃ *cup unsweetened Pineapple Juice*
> 2¹/₄ *teaspoons liquid Sucaryl*
> 3 *pints fresh unsweetened Strawberries (or 6 cups frozen sliced berries, unsweetened)*
> ¹/₄ *teaspoon Vanilla Flavoring*
> ²/₃ *cup granulated Sucaryl*

Beat egg yolks thoroughly in top of a double boiler. Add liquid Sucaryl and vanilla flavoring. Cook over boiling water, beating constantly, until thickened. Add pineapple juice slowly and cook until filling is consistency of whipped cream. Cool.

Fill the cooled crusts with the pineapple sauce and top with strawberries sweetened with granulated Sucaryl.

One serving equals 1 Fruit Exchange, ¹/₂ Meat Exchange.

- - - - - - - - - -

Exchanges for one serving of the entire menu equal 1 A Vegetable, 2 Fruit, ¹/₂ Bread, 4¹/₂ Meat, 3¹/₂ Fat.

* * * * *

SEATED DINNERS

In the hectic rush of complex daily living a seated dinner offers respite and comradeship not to be surpassed. When established as part of a family routine it emphasizes a sense of belonging. When projected for guests it creates a happy approach to gentle living and communion among friends. This is why the small seated dinner is called the highest compliment one can pay when entertaining.

Menus and Recipes for Four

Baked Ham

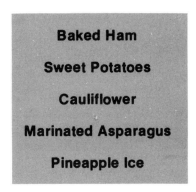

Baked Ham

Sweet Potatoes

Cauliflower

Marinated Asparagus

Pineapple Ice

Baked Ham
(4 servings — 3 ounces ham plus 3 teaspoons sauce, each)

3/4	pound lean cooked Ham, sliced
1¹/₂	teaspoons Flour
1	Egg
1	teaspoon Dry Mustard
¹/₂	cup boiling Water
1	teaspoon Vinegar
1	teaspoon liquid Sucaryl
1	teaspoon Margarine
1	pinch of Salt

Wrap sliced ham in aluminum foil; heat in 200-degree oven for 20 minutes. Beat egg and mix with dry mustard, flour, vinegar, Sucaryl, and salt. Add boiling water. Cook, stirring constantly, until thickened. Remove from stove and add margarine. Serve warm over ham.

One serving equals 3 Meat Exchanges.

Sweet Potatoes (4 servings — ³/₄ cup each)

    3   medium-sized *Sweet Potatoes*
    ¹/₈   teaspoon *Butter Flavoring*
    ¹/₄   teaspoon *Salt*

Wash potatoes and bake in 400-degree oven for 1¹/₄ hours. Remove skins and mash with butter flavoring and salt.
One serving equals 3 Bread Exchanges.

Cauliflower (4 servings — ¹/₄ head each)

    1   small head *Cauliflower*
    4   teaspoons *Margarine*
    1   slice *Bread, crumbled*
    1   teaspoon *Salt*

Steam salted cauliflower whole over small amount of water until tender (about 10 minutes). Brown bread crumbs in margarine. Remove cauliflower to serving dish, cut in quarters, and sprinkle with browned crumbs.
One serving equals 1 A Vegetable Exchange, 1 Fat Exchange.

Marinated Asparagus (4 servings — 4 spears each)

    1   1-pound can *Asparagus Spears*
    Juice of ¹/₂ *Lemon*
    ¹/₄   cup *Cider Vinegar*
    ¹/₂   teaspoon *Seasoned Pepper*
    ¹/₃   teaspoon *liquid Sucaryl*
    ¹/₂   teaspoon *Salt*

Drain asparagus (retaining ¹/₂ cup of juice) and place in covered dish. Mix the retained juice thoroughly with the other ingredients and pour over asparagus. Cover and refrigerate over night.
One serving equals 1 A Vegetable Exchange.

Pineapple Ice (4 servings — ³/₄ cup each)

    2   cups unsweetened canned Pineapple, with Juice
    12   Ice Cubes

Place ingredients in blender on high speed for 2 minutes. Add small amount of liquid Sucaryl if additional sweetness is desired. Serve in chilled sherbet glasses with short straw.
  One serving equals 1 Fruit Exchange.

- - - - - - - - - -

Exchanges for one serving of the entire menu equal 2 A Vegetable, 1 Fruit, 3 Bread, 3 Meat, 1 Fat.

* * * * *

Shrimp Curry

Broiled Grapefruit

Shrimp Curry

Buttered Snow Peas

Sliced Tomatoes - Marinated Cucumber

Baked Apple with Topping

Broiled Grapefruit (4 servings — 1/2 grapefruit each)

    2   medium-sized Grapefruit
    4   teaspoons Brown-Sugar Substitute

Cut grapefruit in half and loosen sections. Put 1 teaspoon sugar substitute on each half and broil until bubbly. Serve hot. *One serving equals 1 Fruit Exchange.*

Shrimp Curry (4 servings — 1 cup each)

    40   medium-sized Shrimp, cooked
    1   medium-sized Onion, chopped fine
    3   tablespoons Margarine
    5   teaspoons Flour
    1/2 teaspoon Curry Powder
    1   cup Chicken Bouillon
    1   cup cooked Rice
    1   cup Milk
    1   teaspoon Lemon Juice
    Salt and Pepper

Sauté onion in margarine. Add flour, salt, and pepper, and cook a few minutes. Stir in bouillon and milk, and cook until thickened. Remove from heat and add rice, shrimp, curry powder, and lemon juice. Turn into casserole and bake in 325-degree oven for $1/2$ hour.

One serving equals $1/4$ Milk Exchange, 1 Bread Exchange, 2 Meat Exchanges.

Buttered Snow Peas (4 servings — $1/2$ cup each)

$1^1/_2$ 10-ounce packages frozen Snow Peas
4 teaspoons Margarine

Cook snow peas according to directions on package. Drain, leaving about 1 tablespoon water on them. Add margarine and stir carefully to avoid breaking the pods.

One serving equals $1/2$ B Vegetable Exchange, 1 Fat Exchange.

Sliced Tomato - Marinated Cucumber (4 servings)

3 medium-sized Tomatoes
4 medium-sized Cucumbers
2 tablespoons Vinegar
2 drops liquid Sucaryl
$1/_8$ teaspoon Salt

Peel and slice cucumbers, put in bowl with broken ice cubes for an hour to crisp. Slice tomatoes and arrange on platter. Mix remaining ingredients and pour over cucumbers. Serve on platter with tomatoes.

One serving equals 1 A Vegetable Exchange.

Baked Apple (4 servings — 1 apple each)

4	medium-sized cooking Apples
1	teaspoon Lemon Juice
4	teaspoons granulated Sucaryl
2	tablespoons Water
1	pinch of Salt
	Cinnamon
²/₃	cup Jane's Topping*

Peel a wide circle around the middle of each apple and remove core. Place in baking dish with tight cover. Put ¹/₄ teaspoon lemon juice and 1 teaspoon granulated Sucaryl on each apple and sprinkle with cinnamon. Cover and bake in 375-degree oven for 1 hour.

Serve with 1 tablespoon of Jane's Topping on each apple.

One serving (apple with topping) equals 1¹/₂ Fruit Exchanges.

- - - - - - - - - -

Exchanges for one serving of the entire menu equal ¹/₄ Milk, 1 A Vegetable, ¹/₂ B Vegetable, 2¹/₂ Fruit, 1 Bread, 2 Meat, 1 Fat.

* * * * *

---

*Use recipe for Jane's Topping given in Part IV (see Index), but cut to one-third the quantities designated.

Chicken Marengo

Chicken Marengo

Brown Rice

Green Salad with Oil and Vinegar Dressing

Carrot Casserole

Minted Pears

Chicken Marengo (4 servings — 1/4 chicken each)

1	2 1/2-pound Fryer, cut in quarters
1	cup canned Tomatoes
3	fresh Tomatoes
1/2	pound Mushrooms
3	tablespoons Cooking Oil
1/2	tablespoon Cornstarch
1/2	cup unsweetened Apple Juice
1	clove Garlic
1/4	teaspoon Sweet Basil
1	pinch Oregano
Parsley	
Salt and Pepper	

Wipe chicken with damp cloth, then rub with salt and pepper. Brown chicken in skillet in hot oil. Turn to simmer, cover, and cook about 30 minutes. Remove chicken and set aside.

Dissolve cornstarch in apple juice, and place in skillet with garlic. Simmer until thickened. Add canned tomatoes, bring to a boil, then add fresh tomatoes, mushrooms, and cooked chicken. Cover and simmer for 15 minutes. Garnish with parsley.

One serving equals 1 A Vegetable Exchange, ½ B Vegetable Exchange, 3 Meat Exchanges, 2 Fat Exchanges.

Brown Rice (4 servings — ½ cup each)

1   cup Brown Rice
2   Bouillon Cubes
2   cups Water

Cook rice as directed on package, using water in which bouillon cubes have been dissolved.

One serving equals 1 Bread Exchange.

Green Salad with Oil and Vinegar Dressing
(4 servings — 1 cup each)

4   cups assorted Salad Greens
8   teaspoons Salad Oil
4   teaspoons Vinegar
Salad Herbs, if desired
Salt and Pepper

Mix oil, vinegar, salt, pepper, and salad herbs (optional). Toss with greens just before serving.

One serving equals 2 A Vegetable Exchanges, 2 Fat Exchanges.

Carrot Casserole (4 servings — 1 cup each)

3   cups cooked Carrots, mashed
4   teaspoons Margarine
1   large Onion, chopped fine
1   Green Pepper, chopped fine
1   tablespoon Flour
Salt and Pepper

Sauté onion and pepper in margarine. Add flour, salt, and pepper, and mix well. Combine with carrots and place in casserole that has been sprayed with PAM; bake in 350-degree oven for 30 minutes.

One serving equals 2 B Vegetable Exchanges, 1 Fat Exchange.

Minted Pears (4 servings — ¹/₂ pear each)

4	canned Pear Halves, water-packed
1	cup fresh Mint Leaves, or Mint Flavoring to taste
1¹/₄	cups Water
1	tablespoon Cornstarch
1	tablespoon Lemon Juice
8	teaspoons liquid Sucaryl
1	small pinch Salt
1	drop Green Food Coloring

Boil mint in 1 cup of water for a few minutes. Cool slightly and strain. Mix cornstarch in ¹/₄ cup of water until dissolved, add to mint juice and bring to a boil. Simmer until mixture thickens slightly. Cool, add lemon juice, Sucaryl, and food coloring. Pour over pear halves and store in refrigerator at least 2 hours. Serve in glass dishes or sherbet glasses. Garnish with sprig of mint, if available.

One serving equals 1 Fruit Exchange.

- - - - - - - - - -

Exchanges for one serving of the entire menu equal 3 A Vegetable, 2¹/₂ B Vegetable, 1 Fruit, 1 Bread, 3 Meat, 5 Fat.

* * * * *

Leg of Lamb

Leg of Lamb

Potato Casserole

Green Peas

Fruit Salad

Mocha Pudding

Leg of Lamb (4 servings — 3 ounces each)

1   *Leg of Lamb, 5 to 6 pounds*
3   *cloves Garlic*
Salt and Pepper

With small knife, pierce outside of leg of lamb all over, at points about 2 inches apart, and insert slivers of garlic. Put lamb on a rack in a broiling pan and insert meat thermometer through the middle of the meat. Roast in 475-degree oven for 30 minutes. Reduce heat to 300 degrees and cook 2 hours longer. Do not put water in broiling pan. Roasting thermometer should indicate 175 degrees for medium, 182 degrees for well done.
One serving equals 3 Meat Exchanges.

Potato Casserole (4 servings — 1 cup each)

> 3   cups Potatoes, peeled and sliced
> 2   cups Carrots, sliced thin
> 1   large Onion, sliced thin
> 2   tablespoons Flour
> 1   tablespoon Margarine
> 2   cups Milk
> 2   teaspoons Salt
> Pepper, if desired
> Paprika

Put alternate layers of potatoes, carrots, and onions in a casserole that has been sprayed with PAM. Sprinkle each layer with a little flour, salt, and pepper. Add milk, dot with margarine, and sprinkle paprika on top. Bake in 350-degree oven for 1 hour.

One serving equals ½ Milk Exchange, 1 B Vegetable Exchange, 1 Bread Exchange, 1 Fat Exchange.

Green Peas (4 servings — ½ cup each)

> 1½   10-ounce packages frozen Green Peas
> 4   teaspoons Margarine

Cook peas according to instructions on package. Drain, leaving a small amount of water in the pan with the peas. Add margarine, and stir.

One serving equals 1 B Vegetable Exchange, 1 Fat Exchange.

Fruit Salad (4 servings — 1 cup each)

> 2   medium-sized Oranges
> 2   dozen Grapes
> 1   cup unsweetened Pineapple Chunks, drained
> 2   small Bananas
> 4   leaves Lettuce

Peel oranges, remove yellow membrane, and cut up sections. Cut grapes in half lengthwise and remove seeds. Toss orange pieces, grapes, and pineapple together and chill. If additional sweetness is desired, add a little granulated Sucaryl. Add sliced bananas at serving time; serve on lettuce leaf.

One serving equals 3 Fruit Exchanges.

Mocha Pudding (4 servings — 1/2 cup each)

2	*tablespoons unsweetened Cocoa*
1	*tablespoon Gelatin*
1	*tablespoon Water*
1 1/2	*cups double-strength Coffee*
1/2	*cup Coffee Cream*
1	*tablespoon liquid Sucaryl*
1/8	*teaspoon Salt*
1	*teaspoon Brandy Flavoring*

Combine gelatin and water. Mix cocoa, salt, and coffee, and bring to a boil. Add gelatin mixture. Cool until syrupy. Fold in Sucaryl, flavoring, and cream. Serve in parfait or sherbet glasses.

One serving equals 1/4 Milk Exchange, 1 Fat Exchange.

- - - - - - - - - -

Exchanges for one serving of the entire menu equal 3/4 Milk, 2 B Vegetable, 3 Fruit, 1 Bread, 3 Meat, 3 Fat.

* * * * *

Roast Beef

Chilled Fruit Soup*

Roast Beef

Pilaf

Broccoli

Vanilla Ice Cream with Fresh Fruit

Chilled Fruit Soup* (4 servings — ³/₄ cup each)

1¹/₃	cups unsweetened Pineapple Juice
1¹/₂	cups Low-Calorie Cranberry Juice
²/₃	cup Water
1¹/₂	tablespoons Tapioca
¹/₂	teaspoon grated Lemon Peel
1	Cinnamon Stick
¹/₄	cup Port Wine
	Liquid Sucaryl

Simmer water and cinnamon stick for about 3 minutes to get essence; remove cinnamon stick. Add tapioca to cinnamon water and cook about 5 minutes, stirring occasionally. Remove from heat and add grated lemon peel. Cool. Add cranberry juice, pineapple juice, and wine. If desired, add liquid Sucaryl. Refrigerate for several hours; serve cold.

One serving equals 2¹/₂ Fruit Exchanges.

*Contains small amount of sugar.

Roast Beef (4 servings—3 ounces each)

> 1   *4-pound Eye-of-the-Round Beef Roast*
> 2   *large Onions*
> 1/2   *cup Water*
> *Salt and Pepper*
> *Accent*

Preheat oven to 350 degrees. Rub meat with salt, pepper, and Accent. Insert meat thermometer into center of roast. Slice onions and distribute on roasting rack. Place meat on top of onions in shallow roasting pan. Add 1/2 cup water and place in oven. Immediately turn oven temperature control down to 200 degrees for the entire cooking period. Add a little water from time to time as needed to keep roast moist. Baste with juices. Cook about 1 hour per pound—until thermometer reaches 140 degrees for rare, 160 degrees for medium, or 170 degrees for well done.

An alternate method of timing the roast, if preparation time is limited, is to cook at 325 degrees for 18 to 20 minutes per pound for rare, 22 to 25 minutes per pound for medium, or 30 minutes per pound for well done. Thermometer readings will be the same as for the slow-cooking method.

Carve into 3-ounce servings.

One serving equals 3 Meat Exchanges.

Pilaf (4 servings—1 cup each)

> 1/2   *cup Vermicelli*
> 1/2   *cup Cracked Wheat*
> 1/2   *cup Long-Grain Rice*
> 2   *tablespoons Cooking Oil*
> 3   *cups Beef Stock, or Bouillon*

Heat oil in heavy skillet and add cracked wheat, rice, and vermicelli. Cook until browned thoroughly, stirring often. Bring

beef stock to a boil. Combine all ingredients in covered baking dish and stir well. Place in 400-degree oven for 25 minutes. Remove from oven and wait 10 minutes before lifting cover.
One serving equals 2 Bread Exchanges, 1½ Fat Exchange.

Broccoli (4 servings—2½ ounces each)

1   *package (10 ounces) frozen Broccoli*
½   *teaspoon Butter Flavoring*
Juice of ½ Lemon

Cook broccoli according to instructions on package. Drain well, saving 2 tablespoons liquid. Add lemon juice and butter flavoring to the liquid, pour over top of broccoli, and serve.
One serving equals 1 A Vegetable Exchange.

Vanilla Ice Cream (4 servings—½ cup each)

Use recipe given in Part IV (see Index).
One serving equals ¾ Milk Exchange.

Fresh Fruit

1   *cup sliced Peaches or Strawberries.*

Serve ¼ cup of fruit over each serving of ice cream.
One serving of fruit equals ½ Fruit Exchange.

- - - - - - - - - -

Exchanges for one serving of the entire menu equal ¾ Milk, 1 A Vegetable, 3 Fruit, 2 Bread, 3 Meat, 1½ Fat.

* * * * *

PART IV

Mix and Match

There is nothing like a change of pace to make meals more interesting.

In the following pages, additional recipes are given for salads, meats, vegetables, desserts, and sauces. Any of these may be substituted for one in like category, i.e., salad, meat, vegetable, or sauce, appearing in Parts I, II, and III, provided, of course, that the bounds of exchanges prescribed by the diabetic's physician are observed.

SALADS

Jellied Beet Salad (6 servings — scant cup each)

1	package D-Zerta Lemon Gelatin
1	tablespoon Vinegar
1	tablespoon granulated Sucaryl
1	16-ounce can diced Beets
¹/₂	cup Celery chopped fine
¹/₂	cup grated Carrots
¹/₂	teaspoon grated Onion
¹/₄	cup finely chopped Green Pepper
1	tablespoon Cream Horseradish

Add enough water to beet juice to make 2 cups. Add vinegar and bring to boil. Add gelatin and stir until dissolved, then mix in horseradish and Sucaryl. Cool until partially thickened; fold in vegetables and pour into molds.

One serving equals 1 B Vegetable Exchange.

Tomato Surprise (8 servings — 3 tomato quarters each)

6	large Tomatoes, quartered
1	large Green Pepper, thinly sliced into rings
1	Red Onion, sliced
³/₄	cup Vinegar
1¹/₂	teaspoons Celery Salt
1¹/₂	teaspoons Mustard Seed
¹/₂	teaspoon Salt
¹/₈	teaspoon Red Pepper
¹/₈	teaspoon Black Pepper
¹/₄	cup cold Water
4¹/₂	teaspoons granulated Sucaryl
1	Cucumber (optional)

Combine vinegar, celery salt, mustard seed, salt, Sucaryl, red and black pepper, and water. Boil rapidly for 1 minute. Pour over tomatoes, green peppers, and onions. Refrigerate. Before serving add peeled sliced cucumber, if desired. Keeps well in refrigerator.

One serving equals 1 A Vegetable Exchange.

Shrimp and Mushroom Salad (4 servings — 1 cup each)

2   cups cooked Shrimp
2   cups sliced raw Mushrooms
1   bunch Watercress
$1/2$ teaspoon crushed Tarragon
8   teaspoons Salad Oil
4   teaspoons Vinegar

Mix oil, vinegar, and tarragon, and pour over mushrooms and shrimp. Marinate 2 to 3 hours. Serve over watercress.

One serving equals 1 A Vegetable Exchange, 1 Meat Exchange, 2 Fat Exchanges.

Sunset Glow Salad (4 servings — 5 ounces each)

1   12-ounce can Apricot Nectar
1   package D-Zerta Lemon Gelatin
1   ounce Lemon Juice
1   can ($8^{3}/_4$ ounces) unsweetened Crushed Pineapple
4   Lettuce Leaves

Dissolve gelatin in $1/2$ cup cold nectar, then add to remaining liquid which has been heated to a boil. Add pineapple and its juice. Chill and serve over leaf of lettuce.

One serving equals 1 Fruit Exchange.

Cherry Tomatoes in Herb Marinade
(10 servings — 4 or 5 tomatoes each)

2	baskets Cherry Tomatoes
2	tablespoons dried minced Onion
1/2	teaspoon Sweet Basil
1/4	teaspoon Black Pepper
1/4	teaspoon Oregano
1	teaspoon Garlic Salt
1/4	cup Red Wine Vinegar
1/4	cup Salad Oil
1/4	cup Olive Oil

Dip tomatoes in boiling water for 20 seconds; rinse in cold water and peel. Combine all other ingredients; pour over tomatoes and chill over night.

One serving equals 1 A Vegetable Exchange, 1½ Fat Exchanges.

Cranberry Salad (4 servings — ½ cup each)

1	cup raw Cranberries
1	small Orange
1	Apple
1	teaspoon Gelatin
2	tablespoons cold Water
2	teaspoons liquid Sucaryl

Do not peel any of the fruit. Wash fruit, remove seeds, and grind all together. Sprinkle gelatin over the water, then warm gently until dissolved. Add gelatin mixture to the ground fruit and pour into mold.

NOTE: This recipe is rather tart, to complement roasted turkey. If more sweetening is desired it may be added.

One serving equals ¾ Fruit Exchange.

Alfalfa Sprouts

Add alfalfa sprouts to your grocery list if you haven't already discovered them. Toss them in any mixture of salad greens for a change of texture and flavor. Try them on sandwiches instead of lettuce.

A sprinkling of alfalfa sprouts on sandwich or salad equals Zero Exchange.

MEATS AND SEAFOOD

Quick Shrimp Curry (6 servings — 1 cup each)

20	medium-sized Shrimp, cooked and cleaned
1	can Condensed Cream of Shrimp Soup
1	tablespoon Margarine
1	cup Sour Cream
3	cups cooked Rice
¹/₂	teaspoon Curry Powder (more if desired)
1	teaspoon Lemon Juice
¹/₂	cup chopped Onion
	Paprika

Cook onion in margarine until tender. Add soup, heat, and stir until smooth. Stir in sour cream and curry powder. Add shrimp and heat again. Sprinkle with paprika and serve over hot rice.

One serving equals ¹/₂ Milk Exchange, 1 Bread Exchange, 1 Meat Exchange.

Veal Parmegiana (6 servings — 1 cutlet each)

6	large Veal Cutlets
2	8-ounce cans Tomato Sauce
1	cup crushed Corn Flakes
2	Eggs, slightly beaten
¹/₃	cup Margarine
¹/₂	cup grated Parmesan Cheese
6	1-ounce slices Mozzarella Cheese
3	drops liquid Sucaryl
1	teaspoon Oregano
¹/₄	teaspoon Onion Salt
³/₄	teaspoon Salt
¹/₈	teaspoon Pepper

Dip cutlets in egg, then in corn flakes. Brown in margarine in skillet. Add 1 tablespoon water, cover, and cook over low heat for 30 minutes, then keep covered and warm. In a saucepan combine tomato sauce, oregano, salt, and Sucaryl, and warm over low heat. Arrange meat in casserole and pour hot sauce over top. Cover with Mozzarella cheese and bake in 400-degree oven until cheese melts (about 20 minutes). Serve with spaghetti.

NOTE: If veal is not available, cube steak may be used.

One serving (without spaghetti) equals 1/2 *Milk Exchange,* 1/2 *B Vegetable Exchange, 4 Meat Exchanges, 2 Fat Exchanges.*

Lasagna (10 servings — 2 cups each)

2¹/₂ pounds lean ground Beef
4   cups creamed Cottage Cheese
5   tablespoons Buttermilk
2   large Eggs
10   cups cooked Wide Noodles
1   can (28-ounce) Italian style Pear Tomatoes
8   Italian Sweet Cooking Peppers
3   tablespoons Tomato Paste
7   medium-sized Onions, chopped
2   teaspoons Sweet Basil
1   teaspoon Italian Seasonings
¹/₂   cup Water
1   teaspoon Cooking Oil
Salt and Pepper
Parmesan Cheese

Brown meat in heavy skillet, then cool. Beat eggs, adding cottage cheese, buttermilk, salt and pepper. Cook noodles according to directions on package, adding 1 teaspoon cooking oil to water for easier handling of noodles. Simmer chopped tomatoes, onions, tomato paste, water, and seasonings for 5 minutes. Add peppers from which stems and membranes have been removed.

In baking dish (approximately 11 by 15 inches in size) assemble, in layers, (1) noodles, (2) meat, (3) egg-and-cheese mixture, (4) tomato-onion-pepper mixture (distributing peppers evenly).

Repeat layers, then sprinkle Parmesan cheese over the top. Bake in 375-degree oven for 45 minutes.

One serving equals ¼ Milk Exchange, 1 A Vegetable Exchange, 2 Bread Exchanges, 4 Meat Exchanges.

Barbecued Brisket (20 servings—3 ounces each)

1	6-pound Brisket Roast
1	18-ounce bottle Cattlemen's Barbecue Sauce
5	ounces Worcestershire Sauce
2	ounces Liquid Smoke

Salt and Pepper
Celery Salt
Onion Salt
Garlic Salt

Mix all seasonings except barbecue sauce. Place meat on a large piece of aluminum foil and pour seasoning mixture over it. Bring up opposite sides of foil, fold together and roll down to form a tight packet; turn ends of foil up to prevent leakage. Refrigerate over night. Then bake in 250-degree oven for 5 hours.

Open foil and pour on ½ bottle of barbecue sauce; return to oven for 30 minutes at 300 degrees. Open foil again and add remaining barbecue sauce; return to oven and cook 30 minutes longer at 300 degrees.

This brisket may be sliced and frozen; it keeps well in a freezer.

One serving equals 3 Meat Exchanges.

Ham Salad (4 servings—⅔ cup each)

1	pound boiled or canned Ham (lean)
8	teaspoons Mayonnaise
4	tablespoons Lemon Juice
4	Lettuce leaves

Chop ham and add mayonnaise that has been mixed with lemon juice. Toss, and serve on lettuce.

One serving equals 4 Meat Exchanges, 1 Fat Exchange.

Molded Shrimp in Aspic (8 servings — $^7/_8$ cup each)

1	pound cooked Shrimp, chopped
4	cups Mixed-Vegetable Juice ("V8" type)
3	ribs Celery, minced fine
1	large Kosher Dill Pickle, chopped fine
1	teaspoon Sweet Basil
2	tablespoons Gelatin

Bring $3^1/_2$ cups vegetable juice to boiling point. Add sweet basil and gelatin that has been softened in $^1/_2$ cup of cold vegetable juice. Chill until almost set, then gently stir in chopped shrimp, celery, and dill pickle.

Sauce for Aspic (8 servings — 3 tablespoons each)

1	cup imitation Sour Cream
$^1/_4$	cup Capers
1	tablespoon Cream Horseradish
2	tablespoons Lemon Juice
$^1/_2$	teaspoon dried Tarragon
1	teaspoon dried Onion Flakes
$^1/_2$	teaspoon Dill Weed

Mix all ingredients and allow to season over night in refrigerator.

One serving of the sauce equals 1 Fat Exchange.

One serving of molded shrimp with *sauce equals 1 A Vegetable Exchange, 1 Meat Exchange, 1 Fat Exchange.*

Pork Chops with Bean Sprouts
(4 servings — 1 chop plus 4 ounces of sprouts each)

> 4   *lean 4-ounce Pork Chops*
> 1   *16-ounce can Bean Sprouts*
> *Salt and Pepper*

Remove fat from chops. Brown chops in skillet; season with salt and pepper. Add small amount of water and simmer for 1 hour. Remove chops to heated platter. Pour off grease from skillet. Add bean sprouts and stir, scraping meat drippings from bottom of skillet. Cook 5 to 7 minutes or until sprouts are crisp, tender, and well seasoned.

One serving equals ¹/₂ A Vegetable Exchange, 2 Meat Exchanges.

VEGETABLES

Sweet-Sour French Green Beans (4 servings — 1/2 cup each)

1   16-ounce can French Green Beans, drained
1/2   cup granulated Sucaryl
1/4   cup Wine Vinegar
3   whole Cloves
1/4   cup Water
1   Cinnamon Stick
1/2   teaspoon Celery Seed
1/2   teaspoon Salt

Combine all ingredients except beans. Bring to a boil. Pour over drained beans. Cool. Cover and refrigerate over night.
One serving equals 1 A Vegetable Exchange.

Best Baked Celery (6 servings — 3/4 cup each)

4   cups finely chopped Celery
1   8-ounce can Water Chestnuts
1/2   cup blanched Almonds, sliced thin
1/4   cup Water
1   cup Chicken Bouillon
1   4-ounce can Pimientos, diced
2   tablespoons Cornstarch
Salt

Cook celery until tender (about 30 minutes) in chicken bouillon. Add salt. Mix cornstarch with water, add to celery, and cook to thicken. Add almonds and pimientos. Pour into casserole that has been sprayed with PAM. Bake in 325-degree oven for 30 minutes.
One serving equals 1 A Vegetable Exchange, 1 Fat Exchange.

Buttered Beets (4 servings — ³/₄ cup each)

8   *medium-sized Beets, fresh*
2   *tablespoons Butter*
Salt and Pepper

Leave about 2 inches of tops on fresh beets to prevent bleeding while cooking. Cover beets with water and boil until tender (about ¹/₂ hour). Remove from fire and cool. Skins will slip off when pressure is applied. Slice into pan, add salt, pepper, and butter; heat thoroughly.

NOTE: *Butter* and *fresh* beets are specified, as butter enhances the superior flavor of fresh beets.

One serving equals 1¹/₂ B Vegetable Exchanges, 1¹/₂ Fat Exchanges.

Broccoli Oriental (4 servings — ⁵/₈ cup each)

2   *10-ounce packages frozen Broccoli*
1   *tablespoon Salad Oil*
1   *tablespoon Vinegar*
1   *tablespoon Soy Sauce*
4   *teaspoons Brown-Sugar Substitute*
2   *tablespoons Sesame Seed*

Cook broccoli according to directions on package; drain. Mix remaining ingredients, bring to a boil, and pour over hot broccoli.

One serving equals 1 A Vegetable Exchange, 1 Fat Exchange.

Broiled Tomato (4 servings — 1 tomato each)

4   *large fresh Tomatoes*
Parmesan Cheese, grated
Salt and Pepper

Slice tops off tomatoes and place tomatoes in broiler pan that has been sprayed with PAM. Sprinkle lightly with cheese and a little salt and pepper. (Bread crumbs may be substituted for cheese, if desired.) Broil until bubbly.

One serving equals 1 A Vegetable Exchange.

Eggplant Casserole (6 servings—1 cup each)

1	large or 2 medium-sized Eggplants
2	large Onions, sliced
¼	cup Margarine
¾	pound fresh Mushrooms, sliced
4	large Tomatoes, chopped
2	Green Peppers, seeded and cut in strips
1	clove Garlic, crushed
2	teaspoons Salt
¼	teaspoon Pepper
1	Bay Leaf
¼	teaspoon Sweet Basil
¼	teaspoon Oregano
⅛	teaspoon Clove
¼	cup dry Bread Crumbs

Peel eggplant, cut in 1-inch slices, cover with boiling water, and simmer for 10 minutes. Drain well. Melt margarine, add onions and garlic, and cook until light brown. Add mushrooms and cook for 5 minutes. Add tomatoes, green pepper, and seasonings; simmer for 10 minutes.

Put alternate layers of eggplant and sauce in casserole that has been sprayed with PAM. Cover with bread crumbs. Bake in preheated 325-degree oven for 1½ hours. Start with casserole covered, but remove lid when about half done.

One serving equals 1 A Vegetable Exchange, 1 B Vegetable Exchange, 2 Fat Exchanges.

Eggplant and Noodles (6 servings—1 cup each)

1	medium-sized Eggplant, peeled and diced
2	cups cooked Noodles
2	cups chopped fresh Tomatoes
1	cup thinly sliced Green Pepper
1/4	cup Flour
1/4	teaspoon Oregano
1/4	teaspoon Sweet Basil
1/4	teaspoon Rosemary
1/2	cup Beef Bouillon
1/2	cup grated sharp Cheddar Cheese
2	tablespoons Margarine
1/2	cup Cracker Crumbs

Salt and Pepper

Place noodles, tomatoes, and green peppers in layers in a 2-quart casserole that has been sprayed with PAM. Sprinkle flour, salt, pepper, oregano, sweet basil, and rosemary over the top. Cover with eggplant. Pour bouillon and melted margarine over the assembly. Top with grated cheese and cracker crumbs. Bake in 300-degree oven for 1 hour.

One serving equals 1 A Vegetable Exchange, 1½ Bread Exchanges, ½ Meat Exchange, 1 Fat Exchange.

Poached Mushrooms and Artichokes
(4 servings—1 cup each)

1	pound fresh Mushrooms, sliced
1	10-ounce package frozen Artichoke Hearts
2	large Tomatoes, peeled and quartered
1	Bermuda Onion, chopped
1/2	Green Pepper, chopped
3/4	cup Sherry Wine
3/4	cup Chicken Broth
1/2	teaspoon Butter Flavoring

Salt

Preheat electric skillet to 230 degrees; pour in wine, broth, and butter flavoring. Add all vegetables and season with salt. Cover and cook until artichokes are done and other vegetables are still crisp (about 15 minutes).

One serving equals 1 A Vegetable Exchange, 1 B Vegetable Exchange.

Think-Thin Stuffed Mushrooms
(2 servings—2 mushrooms each)

4	large fresh Mushrooms
2	ounces Swiss Cheese
1	slice Bread, toasted
2	tablespoons chopped Parsley
1	teaspoon chopped Chives
1	tablespoon Dry Wine

Garlic Powder
Salt and Pepper

Remove stems from mushrooms. Mince stems finely with cheese, bread, parsley, chives, and seasonings, then moisten with wine. Use this mixture to fill mushroom caps. Bake in 325-degree oven for 15 to 20 minutes. Serve hot.

One serving equals ½ Bread Exchange, 1 Meat Exchange.

Onions Stuffed with Spinach (6 servings—1 onion ring each)

1	10-ounce package frozen chopped Spinach
1	3-ounce package Cream Cheese, softened
1	Egg
1	large Flat Onion
¼	cup grated Parmesan Cheese
½	cup soft Bread Crumbs
¼	cup Milk
¼	teaspoon Salt
1	dash of Pepper

Cook spinach according to directions on package; drain well. Beat cream cheese and egg until light. Add bread crumbs, cheese, milk, salt, and pepper; mix well. Stir in drained spinach. Peel onion and cut in half crosswise. Separate layers to form six shells; place shells in a 9- by 9-inch baking dish. Fill in base of shells with small onion pieces, if necessary. Spoon spinach mixture into shells. Cover with aluminum foil and bake in 350-degree oven for 40 minutes.

One serving equals ½ B Vegetable Exchange, 1 Fat Exchange.

Red Cabbage (8 servings — ½ cup each)

1	small head Red Cabbage, shredded
2	small tart Apples, unpeeled, diced
½	cup Cider Vinegar
2	tablespoons Water
3	tablespoons Margarine
1	small pinch Salt
3	tablespoons granulated Sucaryl

Place cabbage, apples, vinegar, water, margarine, and salt in saucepan and cook for about 15 minutes. Remove from heat, add Sucaryl, and toss thoroughly. Serve warm.

One serving equals 1 A Vegetable Exchange, ½ Fruit Exchange, 1 Fat Exchange.

Ginger Carrots (6 servings — ½ cup each)

4	cups Carrots, sliced diagonally
1	cup Orange Juice
½	cup Chicken Broth
3	whole Cloves
¾	teaspoon Ginger
1½	teaspoons grated Lemon Rind
3	tablespoons granulated Sucaryl

Put all ingredients in saucepan and bring to a boil. Cover and simmer for 30 minutes or until carrots are tender.

One serving equals ¹/₂ B Vegetable Exchange, ¹/₂ Fruit Exchange.

Creamed New Potatoes and Peas
(8 servings — ¹/₂ cup each)

1	1-pound can small New Potatoes
2	10-ounce packages frozen Green Peas
1	10¹/₂-ounce can Condensed Cream of Chicken Soup
¹/₄	cup minced Celery

Mix celery with frozen peas and cook according to directions on package as given for peas alone. Add soup and drained potatoes and continue heating until potatoes are hot, stirring frequently.

One serving equals 1 Bread Exchange, ¹/₂ Fat Exchange.

Vegetable Medley (10 servings — 4 ounces each)

1	10-ounce can cut Green Asparagus
1	10-ounce can small Green Peas
1	10-ounce can sliced Mushrooms
¹/₂	teaspoon Butter Flavoring
¹/₂	cup blanched Almonds, sliced
1	4-ounce jar Pimiento strips
¹/₂	cup crushed Bread Crumbs

Spray casserole with PAM. Drain vegetables, saving liquid for later use. Place vegetables in layers in casserole, sprinkling bread crumbs and almonds over each layer. Add butter flavoring to ¹/₄ cup of mixed-vegetable liquids, and pour over layers. Bake in 325-degree oven for 1 hour.

One serving equals 1 A Vegetable Exchange, 1 Fat Exchange.

Ratatouille (4 servings – 1/2 cup each)

2	medium-sized Zucchini
1/2	small Eggplant
1	small Green Pepper
1	medium-sized Onion
1	large Tomato, diced
1	clove Garlic, crushed
1/2	teaspoon Salt
1/2	teaspoon Sweet Basil
3	tablespoons Olive Oil

Cut zucchini and eggplant into 1/2-inch slices and salt lightly. Let stand on paper towels about 15 minutes, then dry with paper towels and place in small casserole. Slice onion and pepper and place these on top of vegetables in the casserole. Drizzle olive oil over contents of casserole. Combine tomato and seasonings and pour over the top. Cover casserole and bake contents in 350-degree oven for 2 hours.

One serving equals 1 A Vegetable Exchange, 2 Fat Exchanges.

Baked Squash (6 servings – 1 cup each)

2	cups cooked Squash (any variety), drained and mashed
1	cup chopped Onions
2	Eggs
2	tablespoons Worcestershire Sauce
1	can Condensed Cream of Mushroom Soup
1	cup Cracker Crumbs
1	cup grated Cheese
	Salt and Pepper

Combine squash, onions, eggs, Worcestershire sauce, cracker crumbs, soup, salt and pepper, and half the cheese. Place in casserole and top with remaining cheese. Bake in 350-degree oven for 30 minutes.

One serving equals 1 B Vegetable Exchange, 1/2 Bread Exchange, 1 Meat Exchange, 1/2 Fat Exchange.

DESSERTS

Apple Pie (from Dried Apples) (8 servings — ¹/₈ pie each)

4   packages dehydrated Apple Snacks (¹/₂ ounce per package)
3   cups Water
¹/₂   teaspoon Cinnamon
¹/₄   cup Flour
³/₄   cup granulated Sucaryl
¹/₂   teaspoon Salt
1   tablespoon Lemon Juice
¹/₄   teaspoon Butter Flavoring
1   unbaked Pie Shell, 9-inch

Simmer apples, lemon juice, and water for 15 minutes. Let cool and add butter flavoring. Mix flour, cinnamon, Sucaryl, and salt; stir into apples. Put mixture into pie shell and bake in 350-degree oven for 20 to 25 minutes. Remove from oven and sprinkle with topping (recipe follows). Return to oven and bake at 325 degrees for 20 minutes, or until topping is slightly browned.

Topping for Pie

3   tablespoons Brown-Sugar Substitute
2   tablespoons Margarine
¹/₈   teaspoon Salt

With fingers, rub together the brown-sugar substitute, margarine, and salt. Sprinkle this over pie.

One serving (pie with topping) equals 1 Fruit Exchange, 1 Bread Exchange, 3 Fat Exchanges.

Apple Turnovers (4 servings — 1 turnover each)

> 4   slices White Bread
> 4   small cooking Apples, peeled and sliced
> 1   teaspoon Lemon Juice
> 1¹/₂ teaspoons unsweetened Cherry Kool-Aid
> 1   cup Water
> 6   teaspoons granulated Sucaryl
> 2   teaspoons Cinnamon

Remove crusts from bread and roll bread very thin with a rolling pin. In a saucepan place apples, lemon juice, Kool-Aid, water, and 2 teaspoons granulated Sucaryl. Cook until apples are tender (about 10 minutes). Remove apples and drain. Put apples in the centers of the bread slices. Fold the bread crosswise in triangles and pinch the edges together firmly to fashion the turnovers. Place turnovers on broiler. Mix cinnamon and 4 teaspoons granulated Sucaryl; sprinkle half of this mixture over the top of the turnovers and broil until lightly browned. Flip the turnovers so that the under side is now up and sprinkle with the remaining cinnamon-Sucaryl mixture, then brown lightly. Serve hot.

One serving equals 1 Fruit Exchange, 1 Bread Exchange.

Stewed Apples (1 serving — ¹/₂ cup)

> 1   package dehydrated Apple Snacks (¹/₂ ounce)
> ¹/₂ cup Water

Simmer apples in water for 15 minutes. Chill. Use for dessert or for breakfast fruit.

One serving equals 1¹/₄ Fruit Exchanges.

Spanish Cream (4 servings — ²/₃ cup each)

2	Eggs, separated
2	cups Milk
1	tablespoon Gelatin
3	teaspoons liquid Sucaryl
1	teaspoon Vanilla or Brandy Flavoring
1	small pinch of Salt

Place all ingredients, except egg whites, in top of double boiler. Cook over boiling water until mixture coats spoon, stirring constantly. Whip egg whites until stiff, and fold into mixture while it is hot. Pour into four sherbet glasses and refrigerate.

One serving equals ¹/₂ Milk Exchange, ¹/₂ Meat Exchange.

Cherry Cream Pie (8 servings — ¹/₈ pie each)

1	cup water-packed Sour Red Cherries
1	cup Cherry Juice
2	Egg Yolks
1¹/₂	tablespoons liquid Sucaryl
2¹/₂	tablespoons Flour
1	tablespoon Margarine
¹/₈	teaspoon Salt
	Red Food Coloring
1	cup Jane's Topping*
1	baked Pie Shell (9-inch)

Drain cherries, saving juice. Beat egg yolks and add Sucaryl; blend in flour and salt. Stir into cherry juice and cook about 10 minutes, or until clear. Add margarine, then add cherries and a few drops of red food coloring. Pour mixture into baked pie shell, and chill. Add Jane's topping and keep chilled until served.

One serving equals 1 Bread Exchange, 3 Fat Exchanges.

*Use recipe for Jane's Topping given in this section (see Index).

Date-Nut Tart (4 servings—1 tart each)

4	slices White Bread, trimmed
8	Dates, chopped fine
4	tablespoons toasted Sunflower Seed
1/4	cup Water
1	tablespoon granulated Sucaryl
1	small pinch of Salt

Preheat oven to 450 degrees. Roll bread very thin with rolling pin and drape into large muffin tins that have been sprayed with PAM. Combine dates, sunflower seed, water, and Sucaryl. Place in bread cups. Put in oven and immediately lower temperature control to 400 degrees. Bake until edges of bread are lightly browned. Remove from oven and sprinkle Sucaryl over tops.

NOTE: 4 tablespoons of raisins may be used instead of dates.

One serving equals 1 Fruit Exchange, 1 Bread Exchange, 1 Fat Exchange.

Frozen Fruit Sticks (8 servings—3/4 cup each)

1	quart Strawberries, unsweetened
1	quart Milk
3	teaspoons liquid Sucaryl
1	teaspoon Vanilla Flavoring
1/4	teaspoon Almond Flavoring
1/8	teaspoon Salt
16	Paper Cups (3-ounce size)
16	Wooden Sticks

Place all ingredients except the last two listed in blender and beat until thoroughly mixed. Pour mixture into paper cups, insert a stick in each, and freeze. When ready to serve, the cup may be peeled off. Two of the frozen sticks make one serving.

One serving equals 1/2 Milk Exchange, 1/2 Fruit Exchange.

Strawberry Pie (8 servings — ¹/₈ pie each)

2	cups diced fresh Strawberries
2	tablespoons liquid Sucaryl
¹/₄	teaspoon Salt
3	tablespoons Cornstarch
1	cup Water
¹/₂	teaspoon Red Food Coloring
1	tablespoon Margarine
1	baked Pie Shell (9-inch)
2	cups Jane's Topping*

Mix Sucaryl, salt, cornstarch, and water. Cook until thick and clear (about 10 minutes). Add margarine. Cool. Add food coloring and sliced berries; mix gently. Pour into baked pie shell and chill. Cover with Jane's topping and keep chilled until served.

NOTE: Boysenberries or dewberries may be used instead of strawberries.

One serving equals ¹/₂ Fruit Exchange, 1 Bread Exchange, 3 Fat Exchanges.

Frozen Banana-Chocolate Sticks (2 servings — 1 stick each)

1	small Banana, peeled and cut in half
3	tablespoons Evaporated Milk
1	teaspoon unsweetened Cocoa
2	teaspoons liquid Sucaryl
¹/₈	teaspoon Vanilla Flavoring
2	Wooden Sticks

Put a stick in each half of the banana and place in freezer for 2 hours. Combine remaining ingredients and heat until dissolved, then cool. When banana is well frozen, remove from freezer and roll in coating mixture. Wrap in aluminum foil or plastic wrap and return to freezer for half an hour or longer.

One serving equals ¹/₂ Milk Exchange, 1 Fruit Exchange.

*Use recipe for Jane's Topping given in this section (see Index).

Ice Cream (8 servings — ¹/₂ cup each)

1¹/₂	teaspoons Gelatin
2	tablespoons Water
2	cups Whole Milk
1	tablespoon Cornstarch
Dash of Salt	
3	Eggs, separated
1	cup Evaporated Milk
2	teaspoons liquid Sucaryl
2¹/₂	teaspoons Vanilla Flavoring

Mix water with gelatin and set aside. Using a small amount of milk, dissolve the cornstarch and salt, then add this to the rest of the milk placed in the top of double boiler. Cook over boiling water 2 or 3 minutes, until mixture has thickened. Beat egg yolks and add to this mixture. Cook 1 minute longer. Remove from heat and add softened gelatin. Mix well. Add evaporated milk, vanilla flavoring, and Sucaryl. Chill in refrigerator.

When mixture is thoroughly cool, beat egg whites until moderately stiff. Fold into chilled mixture and place in freezer trays. Stir three times at intervals during freezing to make the ice cream smoother.

One serving equals ³/₄ Milk Exchange.

Buttermilk Sherbet (6 servings — ¹/₂ cup each)

2	cups Buttermilk
1	tablespoon liquid Sucaryl
1	Egg White
1¹/₂	teaspoons Vanilla Flavoring
1	cup unsweetened Crushed Pineapple

Combine buttermilk, Sucaryl, and pineapple. Pour into a freezing tray and freeze to a mush-like consistency. Remove to a chilled bowl, add egg white and vanilla flavoring, and beat until light and fluffy. Return to tray and freeze until firm.

One serving equals 1 Fruit Exchange.

Jane's Topping (yield—about 2 cups)

1	tablespoon Gelatin
1	cup cold Water
1	cup Cool Whip
¹/₈	teaspoon Salt
³/₄	teaspoon Lemon Juice

Sprinkle gelatin on water, then heat until gelatin is completely dissolved. Remove from heat and cool. Remove Cool Whip from freezer so it will be at room temperature. When gelatin mixture reaches a thick syrupy stage, mix Cool Whip, salt, and lemon juice with it and refrigerate.

This topping may be counted as Zero Exchange only when used in an amount up to ¹/₂ cup per serving.

Meringues (6 servings—1 meringue each)

2	Egg Whites
1	teaspoon liquid Sucaryl
1	teaspoon Vanilla Flavoring
1	small pinch of Salt

Beat egg whites until stiff. Slowly add salt, Sucaryl, and vanilla flavoring, beating constantly. Drop by tablespoons onto a cookie sheet that has been covered with brown paper. With a spoon, shape egg whites into small cups. Pull the edges up to deepen cup. Bake in 250-degree oven for 1 hour. Remove from paper immediately.

The meringues may be filled with ice cream, puddings, or fruits, adding the exchanges for the filling used.

One serving of meringue (without filling) equals Zero Exchange.

SAUCES

Tomato Catchup (yield — about ³/₄ cup)

6	tablespoons Tomato Paste
1¹/₄	cups hot Water
3	tablespoons Vinegar
¹/₂	teaspoon liquid Sucaryl
1	teaspoon Salt
1	pinch Cayenne Pepper
1	pinch Allspice

Mix all ingredients, heat, and simmer for 1 hour.

One serving (2¹/₂ tablespoons) equals 1 B Vegetable Exchange.

Barbecue Sauce (yield — about 1¹/₂ cups)

1	6-ounce can Tomato Paste
1¹/₂	cups hot Water
3	tablespoons Vinegar
¹/₂	teaspoon liquid Sucaryl
1	teaspoon Salt
¹/₄	teaspoon Chili Powder
1	pinch Cayenne Pepper
3	tablespoons Worcestershire Sauce
¹/₂	teaspoon Liquid Smoke
1	teaspoon minced Dried Onion

Mix water and tomato paste in a saucepan. Add remaining ingredients and salt to taste. Simmer for 1 hour. Sauce will be quite thick.

One serving (1¹/₂ ounces) equals ¹/₂ B Vegetable Exchange.

Diet Sour Cream (yield — 1¹/₂ cups)

1	cup Creamed Cottage Cheese
¹/₂	cup Buttermilk
1	teaspoon Lemon Juice
³/₈	teaspoon Salt

Combine all ingredients in blender until completely smooth. Refrigerate in covered jar for at least an hour before serving. Shake well before serving.

Diet sour cream is good for salads or dips, but will not stand up under heat (in soup or on hot dishes) as well as real sour cream.

In the quantities ordinarily used (2 tablespoons or less per serving) the exchange may be considered as zero.

APPENDIX

Nice to Know

To Add Extra Flavor

Lemon and herbs are useful in adding extra flavor to food without increasing food values. Lemon is an excellent flavor fixer. Here are a few ways it can be used:

Dip slices of raw apple in lemon juice not only for flavor, but also to keep the apple slices from turning brown.

Squeeze a few drops of lemon juice over sautéed mushrooms to accent the flavor.

Substitute lemon juice for vinegar in salad dressings for a change of pace.

Try pouring a little lemon juice over broccoli. Nothing else is needed.

To keep white vegetables white, add 1 tablespoon of lemon juice to the water in which they are cooked.

The key to herb cookery is restraint. One-eighth of a teaspoon of dried herbs or one-half a teaspoon of fresh herbs (chopped fine) is usually an adequate amount for a recipe that serves six.

Cooked foods will taste better when herbs are added during the last stages of cooking. Uncooked foods need to be in contact with herbs as long as possible before serving.

Add a gourmet touch to your menus by experimenting. For example, omelets or scrambled eggs assume a different character if you add a pinch of sweet basil, chili powder, dill, marjoram, oregano, sage, thyme, or rosemary. Try them all, one at a time, of course, and see which your family prefers.

A little saffron makes a nice change when you are serving poultry or game birds.

Fruit compotes assume a pleasing freshness when sweet basil or mint is added.

Mix your own salad herbs. For a start, combine marjoram, savory, and tarragon. Remember—a little goes far.

Meld flavors in any casserole, stew, or soup by adding a pinch of curry powder.

Start growing your own herbs—even on a window sill!

Mince onion, or slice it very thin, and soak in salted ice water for an hour to obtain a more delicate flavor.

Tomatoes and sweet basil complement each other.

Oregano and cilantro are musts for Mexican food. For seasoning Italian food, oregano in addition to sweet basil, marjoram, thyme, rosemary, savory, and sage, is used.

For Eye Appeal

Make food as attractive to the eye as possible. Serve it on your "good" china more often. And why not use your best flat ware all the time? You will enjoy it more than your grandchildren will, and it will make your good food taste better.

A large fruit salad will be enhanced when served in a watermelon shell. For individual servings, fruit may be placed in the shell of half a grapefruit, orange, small melon, avocado, or pineapple.

Metric Equivalents

(for Weights and Measures)

Liquid (Volume Measures)

1 Quart	= 4 Cups	= 0.95 Liter		
1 Pint	= 2 Cups	= 0.48 Liter	= 4.8 Deciliters
1/2 Pint	= 1 Cup	= 0.24 Liter	= 2.4 Deciliters
1/4 Pint	= 1 Gill	= 0.12 Liter	= 1.2 Deciliters
2 Tablespoons	= 1 Ounce	= 1/8 Cup	= 0.3 Deciliter
1 Tablespoon	= 1/2 Ounce	= 1/16 Cup	= 0.15 Deciliter
1 Teaspoon	= 1/6 Ounce	= 1/48 Cup	= 0.05 Deciliter

Dry (Weights)

1000 Grams	=	2.2 Pounds	=	35.2 Ounces
500 Grams	=	1.1 Pounds	=	17.6 Ounces
100 Grams	=	0.22 Pound	=	3.5 Ounces
50 Grams	=	0.11 Pound	=	1.76 Ounces
25 Grams	=	0.055 Pound	=	0.88 Ounce
10 Grams	=	0.022 Pound	=	1/3 Ounce
454 Grams	=	1 Pound	=	16 Ounces
227 Grams	=	1/2 Pound	=	8 Ounces
114 Grams	=	1/4 Pound	=	4 Ounces
57 Grams	=	1/8 Pound	=	2 Ounces
28 1/2 Grams	=	1/16 Pound	=	1 Ounce

BIBLIOGRAPHY

Adams, C.: Nutritive Value of American Foods in Common Units. Agriculture Handbook No. 456; Washington, United States Department of Agriculture, 1975.

Bowes, A. De P., and C. F. Church: Food Values of Portions Commonly Used, 12th Ed. Philadelphia, J. B. Lippincott Co., 1977.

Gibbs, J. C.: Using Spices and Herbs. Cooperative Extension Service, University of Arizona; Tucson, Arizona, 1972.

Hardy, M. A.: Just a Pinch of Herbs. Pamphlet of the Pima County (Arizona) Cooperative Extension Service; Tucson, Arizona, 1972.

Robinson, C. H., with M. R. Lawler: Normal and Therapeutic Nutrition, 15th ed. New York, MacMillan Publishing Co., 1977.

Watt, B. K., and A. L. Merrill: Composition of Foods; Agriculture Handbook No. 8, Revised 1975; Washington, United States Department of Agriculture.

Williams, S. R.: Nutrition and Diet Therapy, 3d ed. St. Louis, C. V. Mosby Co., 1977.

Nutritive Value of Foods; Home and Garden Bulletin No. 72; Consumer and Food Economic Research Division, Agricultural Research Service, United States Department of Agriculture, 1977.

INDEX